HOW TO HAVE A

XXX SEX LIFE

HOW TO HAVE A

XXX SEX LIFE

★THE ULTIMATE VIVID GUIDE★

THE VIVID GIRLS
WITH DAN ANDERSON AND MAGGIE BERMAN

10 Regan Books
Celebrating Ten Bestselling Years
An Imprint of HarperCollinsPublishers
www.reganbooks.com

HOW TO HAVE A XXX SEX LIFE. Copyright © 2004 by Vivid Entertainment, LLC.
All rights reserved. Printed in the United States of America. No part of this book may
be used or reproduced in any manner whatsoever without written permission except in
the case of brief quotations embodied in critical articles and reviews. For information
address HarperCollins Publishers Inc., 10 East 53rd Street, New York, NY 10022.

HarperCollins books may be purchased for educational, business, or sales promotional
use. For information please write: Special Markets Department, HarperCollins
Publishers Inc., 10 East 53rd Street, New York, NY 10022.

FIRST EDITION

Designer: Erin Benach

Printed on acid-free paper

Library of Congress Cataloging-in-Publication Data has been applied for.

ISBN 0-06-058147-6

04 05 06 WBC/RRD 10 9 8 7 6 5 4 3 2 1

To the First Amendment, without which this book would not exist.

contents

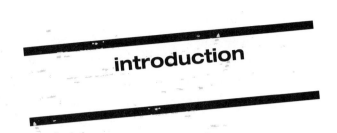

introduction

Before picking up this book, you probably already heard of Vivid Entertainment. The leading producer of adult movies, Vivid is known for their high quality productions that appeal to a broad spectrum of viewers, male and female alike. In addition to Vivid videos, most of which are now distributed in DVD format, the company has grown to include a full range of multimedia products. Riding the crest of a convergence between the new technology and society's increasing candor about sex and sexuality, Vivid operates numerous websites that cater to one's personal tastes, and even offers products ranging from herbal male-enhancement pills to realistic replicas of Vivid Girl body parts. Vivid.com is the primary source of information about Vivid, the Girls, and other products, while Vividdvd.com is the place to visit for the latest DVD releases.

The cornerstone of the company, however, is the movies. The production values are great. Remember the old days of adult movies when you saw the cameraman's shadow across the girl's stomach, or the boom mike creeping down into the shot? You won't see any of that in a Vivid film. And the plots go way beyond the old "come on in, pizza boy" ones of yesteryear. You can even brush up on your literary and film history. Looking for a sexy, suspenseful mix of *The Postman Always Rings Twice* and *Double Indemnity*? Check out *One Way Out*. An updated take on the Greek myth of Phaedra and Hippolytus, where the stepmother falls for her stepson? See *Good Time Girl*. *The Most Beautiful Girl in the World* is a *Faust*-inspired tale in which the devil takes the form of the boss's daughter. Other movies in the Vivid canon are tongue-in-cheek spoofs of common literary conceits. Is your mate leading a secret double life? *So I Married a Porn Star* details one man's realization that his wife's career gives new meaning to the term "layover" when she goes on a business trip. Comedy. Drama. Parody. Suspense. There's a Vivid movie in every genre and one that caters to almost every erotic taste.

One key feature of Vivid movies is that they are meant to be enjoyed by women as well as men. In a modern-day version of the old Hollywood star system, the Vivid Girls are under contract, and work exclusively in Vivid movies. The movies do not exploit women (in fact, it's the women in these movies who often call the shots), they are not violent, and they feature only consensual lovemaking, which includes condoms during intercourse, a Vivid policy. Actor Bobby Vitale says that Vivid treats all of its performers, men and women, with respect. The Vivid Girls have been called the crème de la crème of the industry, but beauty is not the only criterion. "The women we have under contract have to really enjoy what they do. That's very important to us," says Steve Hirsch, the founder and co-chairman of the company.

What is it that makes a Vivid Girl so, well, vivid? First off, they are attractive. Like the glamorous stars from Hollywood's golden age, they are always turned out beautifully. Sure they might walk around the house in a skimpy thong and thigh-highs, but they always do so with flawless makeup and sexy, contemporary hairstyles. Their clothes are sexy, too. Their bodies are slender and toned, but they don't look too skinny. And, perhaps most important of all, the Vivid Girl always gets her man. Once she sets her sights on someone she desires, there's no turning back.

The Vivid Girls are hot, sexy and take charge on-screen. Off-screen, they are bit more like you and me, but, by virtue of what they do for a living, are maybe a little hotter, sexier, and adventurous than most of us. On camera, they live out sexual fantasies every day, and that's what makes them uniquely qualified to offer helpful hints and insider advice to the rest of the world.

"Watching an adult film can be a learning experience, because it gives you new ways to look at the things you do in bed," says Vivid Girl Jenna Jameson. Adult movies offer a glimpse into a world where attitudes toward sex, the approach to the sexual act, and the creativity brought to bear on erotic action are all on a more intense level than most people experience in their everyday lives.

This book is about taking your own sex life to a higher level, to a place where inhibitions fall away and creativity and a sense of adventure flourish. The adult world's top male and female stars, and their directors, offer their expertise, of both their on-camera exploits and their private bedroom discoveries. They share not only techni-

HOW TO BE MORE LIKE A VIVID GIRL

- Always wear six inch heels, even when you are vacuuming, and never take them off during sex.
- Never wear underwear. If you do, then it should be a thong, and it is worn alone, with no clothes on top.
- Never leave the house without making sure your eyelashes are curled, your lipstick is fresh, and your hair falls in that perfectly-mussed-up-but-not-too-messy way.
- Get a French manicure.
- Keep a French maid's uniform handy.
- Show cleavage.
- Change your name to something exotic, like Delicia, or Soleil.
- Don't be afraid to take the lead.

cal tips, but also advice on freeing yourself of the guilt and inhibitions that prevent many of us from fully enjoying ourselves sexually. Go behind the scenes, and step into a world where sex can be as free and unencumbered as it appears in movies.

One of the challenges adult movie directors face is the same one every couple eventually faces: how to keep the action interesting. Many of the tricks used by actors and directors can also be applied in private, including changing your expectations, creating exciting new sexual scenarios, and incorporating the element of fantasy into your sex life. In addition, of course, are all the staples of today's adult movies: exciting positions, unique techniques, and steamy couplings. Whether you want to improve your oral sex skills, bring toys to bed, or simply try out a new position, the Vivid panel of experts is here to help make your erotic productions the award-winning creations they deserve to be. The advice offered encompasses many different situations and possibilities. Some is aimed toward women, some toward men, and some toward couples. Whatever your circumstances, you will find a wealth of useful knowledge. We begin with the basics: communication, seduction, setting the scene. Then we move on to specific technical tips, all accompanied by references for further research. By the end of the book, you might be ready for more "advanced" techniques, so we offer sections on multiple orgasms, multiple partners, anal sex, and more. Whatever you choose to use, or leave to the realm of fantasy, all of it is designed to help you—and your partner, if you have one—have the most satisfying sex ever. So if you're ready to begin, let's get rolling.

1
porn primer

Fantasy File:

He glances over from the bed and sees her in the bath-tub, this beautiful, exotic woman he only met three days before. She looked really good dancing in that strip club, and she looks even better in his apartment. She feels his stare and caresses her breasts as she smiles back at him. She rises from her bath and begins humming a little song. She keeps her eyes on him as she continues to massage her breasts, thighs, and stomach. She playfully picks up a hairbrush and uses it as a microphone for a moment, then rubs it across her silky skin, too. She comes closer—just to the doorway into the bedroom—and jettisons her hairbrush in favor of a gel toy. From the bed, now fully erect just from watching, he tells her to put the toy inside herself. She moistens it in her mouth, then inserts it into her body, pushing it in and out in long, slow strokes. "You like to watch, don't you?" she asks. She turns around, offering him a different view of her auto-erotic exhibition. He strokes his penis in anticipation of feeling her large sensuous lips on him. She crosses the room, takes a sip from her wineglass, and slowly inserts his entire shaft into her mouth. The warm, wet sensation makes him throw back his head in pleasure. He caresses her hair as he whispers, "Yes, that's it, baby, take it all." His penis grows bigger and harder with each motion. As she teasingly licks and kisses the head of his penis, she massages her breast with her other hand and brushes her nipple against his leg.

Next, she lies on her back with her legs in the air as he

begins to enter. When he does, she squeals slightly at the first touch of his hardness and size. He shifts both her legs to the side as he starts to pump faster and faster. With each thrust, he quivers slightly as he feels himself inside her. He keeps going faster and faster. Raising her arms up over her head, she braces herself against the headboard as he continues. Beads of sweat form across his face and chest as he pushes harder and harder into her. "You like that, baby?" he asks in a hoarse whisper. "Yes, yes" is all she can reply. Soon, rocking back and forth with pleasure, she exclaims, "I'm going to come." He wants her to come. As he thrusts into her, he gently massages her clitoris with the tips of his fingers. She feels him everywhere and all around her; her body quivers as she senses her orgasm growing inside, pressing on towards its full release. She squeals again, then moans in sheer ecstasy as the waves of pleasure emerge from deep inside her. He feels her muscles twitching slightly out of control, which makes him even harder and bigger. Her body rocks as she climaxes. Hot, sweating and aroused beyond his dreams, he increases the pace of his thrusts even more, anticipating his own orgasm soon to come . . .

★★ *from* So I Married a Porn Star,
directed by Paul Thomas

Like tech stocks in the nineties, porn is the new hot topic. Everyone seems to be watching it; Jay Leno jokes about it on *The Tonight Show.* Everybody knows who Vivid star Jenna Jameson is, and the first prime-time TV series about a porn king recently aired on Fox. In this new age of sexual openness, men discuss their latest porno acquisitions as freely as they discuss *The Matrix.* And women have gotten in on the act as well. They may not be watching as much as men, but many women have become porn aficionados themselves, joining amateur strip clubs and striptease classes at the local gym, and wearing fashions that are obviously inspired by sex workers and the porn industry. Now women assume that most of the men in their lives spend at least a portion of the day viewing porn online. The easy accessibility of Internet adult entertainment has turned us into a nation of part-time porn buffs.

Of course all this is nothing new. Throughout history, erotic images have found their way into daily life. A quick look at the Greek vases in a major metropolitan museum reveals more than a few giant hard-ons among the satyrs chasing the lovely young maidens. An intriguing wall painting outside Pompeii has perplexed art historians for centuries: the Villa of the Mysteries, as it has been called, features a woman with a whip who looks an awful lot like a dominatrix. Even the Bible has Sodom and Gomorrah, while the Japanese have entertained themselves with erotic "pillow books" through the ages. Literature, too, is full of sexually charged writing. The works of the Marquis de Sade come quickly to mind, but others, such as those by Henry Miller and Anaïs Nin, are equally well known for their erotic content. The joy of sex, in other words, always finds an outlet for expression.

It's practically a truism to say that men are more visual than women when it comes to sex. What we mean by that is that men respond to images more readily than women, who usually favor a story line. But maybe the truth is that we only think that because guys get erections and girls don't. Nowadays, women are as likely to get turned on by a guy in a razor ad as men are by the girls in a beer ad. In any

VIVID GIRL FAVORITES:

WHAT'S THE SEXIEST PART OF A MAN?

Mercedez: His lips and his voice are sexy. I like looking at his lips even more than having them all over me.

Briana: I like the back, shoulders—broad shoulders. I also like a guy's chest.

Sunrise: His back—a well-shaped back. I love big, broad, muscular backs. You can see every muscle move and shift.

Savanna: I like that muscle that goes from the hip bone down to the groin on either side. But it's not so much a physical thing. I like a man's voice, and the way he stimulates me mentally; the way he uses it to arouse me. Not everyone looks like Jean-Claude Van Damme!

Kira: It's got to be the total package!

case, from pinup calendars at the service station to pilfered Victoria's Secret catalogs, we all know that men will take their visuals almost anywhere they can. And it doesn't take much more than that to get a woody. Beyond the visual stimulation, there's a built-in fantasy element every time a guy opens up to the *Playboy* centerfold or surfs into an adult website. Even if just for a second, he imagines the possibility of an encounter with the girl in the picture. And it's that hint of possibility that makes porn so popular.

No longer thought to be the province of perverts in peep booths, porn is increasingly enjoyed by both men and women. For today's sexually liberated woman, porn is just one more tool in her arsenal of personal pleasure enhancers. The men have great bodies and great dicks and they love to show them off, so why shouldn't a girl sneak a peek every now and then? For men, a similar scenario applies: buxom babes who are up for almost anything can be a great way to end the day. As people become increasingly comfortable with porn in their daily lives, more and more couples are watching it together. Again, the fantasy element is key. The couple may not want to actually do everything they see on film, but they can fantasize about it while making love with their partner. As we noted in the introduction, porn is a world where inhibitions are erased. Simply seeing people on-screen behaving in such a liberated way helps many people overcome some of their own fears and issues. As Vivid actor Bobby Vitale puts it, "We're in the happiness business where we give people pleasure by them watching, whether it's lonely guys, or couples, whatever the case may be."

Properly introduced, porn can be a great way to find an interesting new position or pick up a new sex trick. Many people have tried something in bed that they first saw on video, often with good results. In fact, most Vivid DVDs have a section called "Positions Room," which shows short clips of all the examples of a particular position from that particular film. It's a great way to preview a new position you've been wanting to try out with your partner. Not sure how to do a "Reverse Cowgirl"? Head to the Positions Room to find out more. Ditto for blow jobs and cunnilingus. If you're a guy looking to improve his oral skills, check out some girl-on-girl action. Who better to learn from than someone who knows firsthand what it feels like?

It's important to keep in mind that, in real life, not every sexual experience will be "porn-grade" quality. But for those looking to expand their regular repertoire, the DVD can be a great place to start. As one young woman explained in a recent *New York* magazine article, the few sexual experiences she's had with guys who don't look at porn haven't been very good.

❝ ❝ Watching an adult movie is a great aid to any relationship. No matter what, sex will become stale in a relationship. You always have to try new things, and you can see lots of new things in adult movies which may open your mind. ❞ ❞

—Justin Sterling, director

So you want to watch a video with your partner, but you're not sure how to go about it. One way to get started is to let the other person choose the film. That way, they won't feel as though they've had no say in what the evening's activities include. There is a huge variety to choose from, including features made specifically for couples. These tend to feature strong story lines, characters, and production values; moreover, the characters are often married and their lives look a lot like any other couple's. In other words, the characters are ones that almost any couple can relate to on some level, and they could be just the ticket to spicing up a routine sex life.

> **" When couples have problems . . . they can pop in a film and get renewed, they can add to their lives, and maybe release something that they can live through the fantasy. "**
>
> —*Sunrise Adams*

For a woman's point of view, look for movies directed by current and former female stars such as Jenna Jameson, Nina Hartley, Veronica Hart, Candida Royalle, or Jill Kelly. For those who'd rather skip the story and get straight to the sex, check out the wall-to-wall and gonzo sections at the video store.

Don't forget, you need not always leave the house to find good adult movies. For stories with less hard-core content, you can tune into cable channels such as Cinemax, Playboy TV, and the Spice Network. In the world of adult entertainment, there truly is something for everyone, from oral sex fans and anal aficionados to spanking and foot fetishists. Perhaps the best way to find what you want is good old word of mouth: ask a friend for a recommendation. If you can't handle that, then check out the movie reviews on many of the adult websites. Good Vibrations, a sex-toy store in San Francisco that also runs a large catalog operation, prides itself on its thoughtful, in-depth reviews. For the more intrepid, a trip to the video store is in order. Just be prepared to spend some time there, as the number of choices can be overwhelming. One last piece of advice: always rent more than one. That way, the odds of finding at least one scene you like are that much greater.

So the movie's all queued up and ready to go; and you and your partner are raring to go. Pick a position that interests you, pause the video, and then reenact the position. Take turns with the remote control and fast-forward to your favorite parts, then press stop and focus on each other. Touching, massaging, and licking your partner while watching a video can be a great form of foreplay. Then, when you can't stand it any longer, roll over and start directing your own sex scene. You can even leave the video on in the background: the moans and groans of the performers can be the sound track to your own evening of ecstasy.

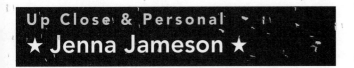

Up Close & Personal
★ Jenna Jameson ★

Rolling Stone magazine has called Jenna Jameson "the woman who put the 'star' in porn star." The adult industry's leading trade journal, *AVN* (*Adult Video News*), named her the top female adult star of all time. Jenna burst onto the adult movie scene in the mid-1990s and won every major award available to a porn actress, the first ever to capture three of the top adult movie awards in the same year. "Once I made up my mind to go into movies," she says, "I wanted to be the most famous, most successful adult star ever." At that she has succeeded, not only through her jaw-dropping performances in adult movies, but also with her numerous appearances in mainstream entertainment sectors.

Born in Las Vegas, Jenna studied ballet as a child. She was a self-described nerd in high school and didn't even have a date to her high school prom. But by her late teens she had blossomed into a voluptuous and sultry stunner with an innocent look. Jenna began getting jobs as a model and topless dancer on the Vegas strip. Before long she was dancing at the world-famous Crazy Horse II, and then *Penthouse* and *Hustler* magazines discovered her and ran pictorials. Since then, she has won virtually every honor the adult industry bestows.

Jenna is a go-getter, in life and in the bedroom. Not satisfied to just lie back in front of the camera, she was infamous in the adult industry for her arguments with directors. "I was always trying to make the movies better," she says. "I couldn't understand why anyone would settle for less. I wouldn't settle for less and didn't think the audience should have to either!" Her perseverance paid off with not only great movies and top sales, but also critical acclaim and armloads of awards from video and trade associations, including a recent Lifetime Achievement Award from *AVN*.

One of the directors she used to clash with was Justin Sterling. "I thought she was a brat," he says of her, while she insists, "I thought he was arrogant." But after a few years, their antagonism turned to attraction. They are now partners in both life and business.

Jenna now runs her own production company, and produces her own movies for *Vivid Video*, with the features directed by her husband, Justin.

Along with a packed schedule of movies, television acting roles, personal appearances, and modeling, the dynamic Jenna is also CEO of ClubJenna, Inc., a fast-growing Internet management, production, and licensing company.

The first feature movie she herself helped produce, *Briana Loves Jenna*, immediately soared to the top of the charts and was named by *AVN* as the top selling and renting video of 2002. *I Dream of Jenna* eclipsed the first release in both VHS and DVD sales and rentals. Her eagerly awaited remake of the movie *The Masseuse* is scheduled for release in 2004.

Jenna's mainstream TV and movie work includes feature roles in Howard Stern's film hit *Private Parts;* the indie horror film *Samhain;* Comedy Central's first feature film, *Porn 'n Chicken;* hosting E! Entertainment TV's *Wild On* series; and a recurring role in the NBC drama *Mr. Sterling.* Jenna has had roles in music videos by Eminem and KORN and makes regular appearances on national television. Her stunning looks have fascinated magazine editors since the start of her career and she has graced over three hundred magazine covers and been featured on more than a thousand magazine articles or in pictorials in *Glamour, Marie Claire, Cosmopolitan, Allure, Jane, Rolling Stone, Revolver, Esquire, Playboy,* and *Penthouse.* She writes regular columns for the British, German, and American editions of *FHM,* a magazine that consistently ranks her as one of the hundred most beautiful and sexy women in the world.

Jenna's climb to the top of the adult movie world has paralleled her internal journey to understanding her own sexual power and freedom. "Women are more inhibited about sex than they have to be," she says. "Maybe it was because I was raised by my father, who was a cop, that I have this no-nonsense attitude about sex. Guys are straightforward about sex and women can be, too." One of Jenna's goals was to produce porn that was as well liked by women as by men. "I think women see my movies, and see my interviews, and think, 'Gee, she's not so different from me.' I hope they realize they can go out and grab what they want just the way I have."

For Jenna, sex is still a magical and wonderful thing. "The moment I usually remember most out of an erotic evening is my orgasm, and how well my partner made me come. It's not very difficult to get me there—I'm very vocal with telling someone exactly what they need to do. If a man can keep me going, that's definitely what sticks in my mind."

And how many times does Jenna come in a typical erotic evening? "That all depends on the session and how tired I am. Sometimes I just want one orgasm and then I'm done, but in my perfect fantasy I think four or five times is wonderful. After that, every muscle is quivering and I am just spent."

Jenna keeps "in shape" by masturbating when the urge strikes. "It's a staple of my day. It's a great stress reliever—at least once a day. And it shouldn't take that long—if you have the right vibrator, it should only take a couple of minutes! I think it's important to do it as much as possible. It puts you in tune with your own body and helps you convey to your lover what you want them to do. How are you going to expect your lover to do it if you can't do it yourself?"

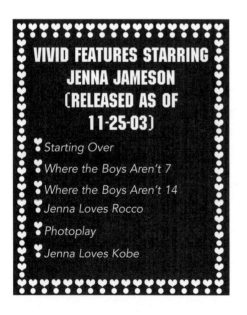

VIVID FEATURES STARRING JENNA JAMESON (RELEASED AS OF 11-25-03)

❣ Starting Over
❣ Where the Boys Aren't 7
❣ Where the Boys Aren't 14
❣ Jenna Loves Rocco
❣ Photoplay
❣ Jenna Loves Kobe

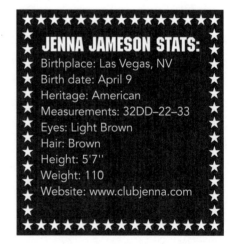

JENNA JAMESON STATS:
★ Birthplace: Las Vegas, NV
★ Birth date: April 9
★ Heritage: American
★ Measurements: 32DD–22–33
★ Eyes: Light Brown
★ Hair: Brown
★ Height: 5'7"
★ Weight: 110
★ Website: www.clubjenna.com

2
preproduction

Fantasy File:

It was a sultry summer night, a real scorcher, and the downstairs dressing room they shared was hotter than hell. "I hope the air-conditioning is cranked up really high tonight," she says as a single bead of sweat trickles down her chest to the glistening valley between her breasts. "You can say that again," answers the buxom blonde who fixes her hair and applies the last of her stage makeup at the other table. As they adjust the pièce de résistance of their identical costumes, the black-and-red patent-leather opera-length gloves custom-made to match their thigh-high stiletto boots and bustiers, someone knocks on the door. "Five minutes to showtime," says the voice, barely audible over the pulsating sounds of the music upstairs. They glance at each other for a moment, and then each sees the reflection of herself in the stage mirrors on opposite walls of the small room. For a moment, it's like seeing double, a multiplication of beautiful blondness repeated into infinity. People often took them for sisters, twins, in fact, with their similar heights and bodies, refined features, and most conspicuously, their massive matching manes of long blond hair. Now, after performing their act together for some time, they even move like each other, the same sexy jut of the hip, the swaying walk, and the "I know I look hot" attitude that makes them so popular with the club's patrons. What most people didn't know was that their relationship is closer than that between any sisters. "It's showtime," says Janine. "Let's go and light those guys on fire tonight."

The DJ changes the music, signaling their introduction. As they step through the curtain onto the stage, they sense by the noise level that many of the guys in the room have cooled themselves off with more than the usual number of beers and cocktails for a Thursday night. This particular gentlemen's club attracts a pretty diverse crowd, including young guys out with their buddies for a night of male bonding and sexy entertainment, as well as a sprinkling of businessmen stopping by after a late night at the office. Maybe it's the heat, but tonight the men seem louder, more anxious, and hungrier for action than usual.

Julia and Janine parade their assets around the stage so the guys can take it all in. It is an image of a fantasy almost too glamorous to be true. Two gorgeous blondes, flamboyantly decked out in provocative black-and-red costumes, complete with silver studs, flowing capes, and snap-off straps in all the right places. The girls position themselves with Julia's back and ass pressed up against Janine's front side. Together, they do a slow bump and grind to the driving rock beat, which, they know, is raising the excitement level up a notch. The crowd claps as one girl forcefully puts her arm around the other, holding her in a headlock. Then, as they both crouch down, letting their cleavage spill out so the guys in the audience get a good glimpse, Janine draws in close behind Julia, sniffing her from behind like a bitch in heat. This is no ordinary strip show. There's definitely something primal, almost animal, about the whole routine, and it's obvious the girls are getting off on the power of their own exhibitionist performance. Not only are they the objects of all the male lust and desire in the room, but there is also an undeniable, powerful electricity between the two of them.

The guys hoot and cheer as Janine forcefully grabs Julia by the hair and turns her head around. She forces Julia down to a kneeling position, pushes her face deep into the hot V between her legs. As she grinds to the music, she thrusts her pussy into Julia's angelic face. Janine smiles as she eyes two guys up front, close to the stage, massaging their burgeoning hard-ons.

For their second scene, both girls strip everything off except their shiny, high-heeled boots, exposing their breasts, asses, and pussies without constraint. They slowly circle around each other on all fours, cautiously sniffing each other like animals. Janine locks Julia's arm and carefully lowers her down onto her back. Moving her own hips in and out in time with the music, she clutches Julia's pussy and lifts her pelvis up and down off the floor. Then, with theatrical precision, Janine spreads her legs wide for Julia to come up, eagerly stroking Janine's pussy. Tongues extended, the girls give each other a long, wet kiss and hold on tightly as they simulate the urgent thrusting motions of sex. The guys really go wild with the image of two gorgeous blondes sexing it up and roughing it up with each other. Meanwhile, both girls know down deep inside that their well-choreographed striptease act has excited more than just the guys.

The crowd can almost smell the heady mix of female aromas as Janine positions Julia in full view and teasingly licks her bare pussy. Defiantly, she leads Julia around in a circle, holding on to her long, wild mane like a leash, or like an animal trainer putting a show dog through its paces. Julia moves on all fours like a magnificent wild and noble creature that has been captured and tamed. Getting down low, they writhe around on the stage, heads back, lips parted, ecstatic. Clearly, Janine is in charge. And then, almost to demonstrate the master's power over a slave, Janine seizes a candle and drips hot wax slowly down Julia's back and into her ass crack. The crowd is mesmerized. Then it's Julia's turn. She pours a stream of wax down her belly so that the last drop stops and hardens on the opening of her pussy slit. As

the men in the audience clap and cheer to signal their ap-
proval, the girls caress each other tenderly and kiss sweetly.

Naked, back in their dressing room after the show, Janine jokingly asks, "Was it good for you?" Without hesitation, Julia smiles and innocently pulls out the wad of bills
that one man, Trey Williams, had placed in her boot during
the performance. "It pays to show a guy a little attention,"
she says to Janine, who, for a split second, shows just the
slightest twinge of jealousy. Just then, one of the stage-
hands knocks on the door and delivers an expensive magnum of champagne. The note confirms that it's a gift to Julia
from the admiring Trey. Rather than falling into the role of an
envious, suspicious lover, Janine suggests they open the
bottle to celebrate. "What shall we drink to?" asks Julia. "To
us," answers Janine. And with that, Janine puts the cold bottle between her thighs, pops the cork, and sprays the cool,
bubbly fluid all over the two of them. It feels great on their
hot, sweaty bodies and tired muscles. Shaking the bottle up,
Janine shoots more liquid onto Julia and begins to massage
and lick the dripping champagne off her now hardened nipple. And, without another word, the voluptuous blondes begin working their wet, eager tongues all over each other.

★★ Blondage,
directed by Toni English

What's So Special About Porn Stars?

The way most people initially think about porn stars is not so different from the way they think about fashion models. Both have become
dazzling media figures in today's pop culture. Of course, there are
some models who might appear daily in newspaper ads, but no one
really recognizes them or knows their names. And then there are the
supermodels who have their own fan clubs and websites, and who are
invited to host TV shows and attend all sorts of glamorous events. It's

the same way with adult movie stars, and the Vivid Girls are the supermodels of porn.

But beyond this, there are certain porn stars as well as models who are lucky enough to possess the special combination of a beautiful face, a great body, and the ability to project the essence of "the girl next door." In other words, they are pretty, sweet, and very, very sexy without seeming trashy. These girls are the ones who grace the pages of the Victoria's Secret catalog, the *Sports Illustrated* swimsuit issue, and, of course, appear in Vivid films. It is these types to whom women can easily relate, and whom guys tend to fantasize about. And that's exactly what makes them so attractive.

Like fashion models, adult movie stars are selected because they can portray a "product" in the best possible light. But in this case, the product is sex rather than clothing. And since so much of one's enjoyment of porn films is based on fantasy, most of the actors and actresses who star in these films are the ones who can show off the product to its very best advantage. In other words, they are mostly young, good-looking men and women with attractive faces, great bodies, and ample endowments. Let's face it: most people would rather fantasize about having sex with someone who looks and feels great than with the office geek in the next cubicle. And that's what porn stars are all about. They represent ideal images of the hottest, sexiest, and most willing lovemaking partners one can possibly imagine; an erotic fantasy one can enjoy alone or with someone else in the privacy of their own home.

Clean Up

Naturally, not everyone is graced with the near-perfect faces and sexy, toned bodies of porn stars. But even some of the stars would look a lot worse if they didn't pay attention to the impeccable hygiene and grooming that are required on the set. Here are a few tips.

It goes without saying that the first order of business for men and women alike is to make sure you and whatever clothing you're wearing smells fresh, and that your body is squeaky-clean. Most people like the subtle, sexy scent emitted by the opposite sex. But no one wants to be memorable because of overpowering body odors under the arms, around the privates, or on stale articles of clothing. There is no doubt about it; the cleaner you are the more desirable you are. Show some respect for your costar, and clean up your act.

And while we're on the subject of odors, in some movies, such as *The Audition,* one of the girls puts special scents on her breasts and elsewhere. On the set, it's preferable to be fragrance-free so that one's costar doesn't start sneezing in the middle of a scene. But in your private productions, you can use your partner's favorite scent in a few well-placed spots, which they will associate with you forever.

Nail It

The next order of business, again for both sexes, is to make sure your nails are clean, well trimmed, and manicured. In certain films, like *Bangkok Nights,* a Vivid actress might have long, red dragon lady nails because of the special character she is playing. But this is an effect to enhance the story line and mood of that movie. No one relishes the thought of scraggly or extra long nails probing an orifice because they can do some real damage. You'll notice in most adult productions, every girl has extremely well-manicured nails, and the guys' nails are clean as well. Vivid Girl Sunrise Adams puts it plainly. "I don't like [dirty] fingers inside of me," she says. "I worry about the stuff under their nails."

Bare Essentials

Shaving and waxing have somewhat different implications for men and women.

No woman wants her face all red and sore because the guy she was kissing forgot to shave. Men's facial hair is usually pretty coarse, so it's important to shave, or to keep beards and mustaches well groomed. And speaking of sensitivity, one important tip for guys comes from Vivid Girl Tawny Roberts. "I don't like it when men are scruffy, so please shave before a bedtime date. We're tender down there! Smooth skin obviously feels better than rough stubble."

Speaking of stubble, you've probably seen a lot of different pubic grooming options in adult movies. In most of the recent Vivid releases, the women's pubic areas are often bare. But in slightly older movies, like *Suite 18, Lotus,* and others, many of the women have neatly trimmed and shaped pubic areas. Some of this is just the style of the times. A few years ago, it was considered au courant for a woman to style her pubic hair into a small strip, a neat minitriangle, or even into something fun, like a heart. A bikini wax meant merely removing stray hair around the mound or near the buttocks—hair that shouldn't peek out of a swimsuit. More recently, however, the popular trend has been toward the Brazilian bikini wax, which takes everything off from the front all the way around to the back. Vivid Girl Kira Kener suggests, "Go and get waxed. It's fast, it's easy, it leaves it so smooth, and you don't have to worry about it for a while." If you prefer this look, we suggest leaving it to a professional rather than trying to do it at home. But during filming, a clean sweep gives the camera person terrific close-up shots.

Sometimes women groom for aesthetics and because they like the way it looks, but it can also heighten a woman's sensitivity during oral sex. Vivid Girl Dasha says, "It feels ten times better to have a guy go down on you when you are shaved." Yet some guys like a little bit of hair because it captures the special fragrance that a woman gives off when she's aroused. If you prefer a natural look, then we still recommend a good trim, especially on your vaginal lips. An electric beard trimmer will give you a closer cut than scissors, without leaving you completely hairless. This will make the area neater and easier for him to navigate.

If you want to go completely bare, you have a few options. Shaving is the easiest and least expensive. Vivid Girl Mercedez says, "I shave the morning of a scene. If I shave the night before, I could wake up with a little stubble. I use tweezers to get out the ingrown hairs." And Sunrise adds, "I do it every day. I use skin tone Clearasil afterward to prevent ingrown hairs. And if my skin is really chafed or raw from too much sex, I use Neosporin. It really helps you heal; I have it in every drawer of my house."

You should shave during or after a shower or bath, once warm water has softened the skin. Tawny shaves every other morning in the shower. "The more I shave, the less likely I am to have bumps or other problems." And always use shaving cream and a fresh razor. Rinse the freshly shaved area with cool water to help soothe the skin and close pores. You may want to wear boxer shorts, "boy-cut" underwear, or no panties for a day or two to avoid irritating the delicate bikini line with the elastic of your undies.

Guys might cringe at the thought of shaving or waxing their private parts, but in today's adult movie industry, you see it quite often. Male porn stars like to have that area bare for several reasons. First, it looks clean and neat on film. Second, it makes their genitals stand out and even look a bit bigger. When two guys are shooting a threesome with a girl, they usually match each other and go smooth. A good example of this is the locker-room scene in *Student Body,* where Dasha and two football players go at it in all sorts of positions. Everyone is as hairless down there as a newborn.

Most guys prefer to shave because they're used to shaving their faces, and they have all the stuff they need to do it on hand. They especially prefer shaving their balls rather than waxing because the testicle area is supersensitive. Other guys do a combination of shaving their balls and waxing the pubic and anal areas—especially if the script calls for some rimming action.

Naked or Not?

66 I like to leave on my beautiful bra and panties, and I let him take them off. You have to let him see it! What's the point if you take it right off? It's fun to leave on thigh high stockings, too. 99

—*Savanna Samson*

It's rare to see a totally nude star in a porn film because that somewhat undone, nude-but-not-quite-naked look is eminently more erotic than being completely in the buff. Why? Well, first, it's like the peekaboo game; it keeps them guessing about what's hiding underneath and what might pop out next. Second, there are just some articles of clothing that look really sexy on women, like garter belts, thongs, push-up bras, tight sweaters, and stiletto boots. "In my private life I slip into sweatpants and sneakers," says Dasha. "But when we go out, it's sexy jeans."

In the same vein, undressing is part of getting relaxed and comfortable with each other, and what you are wearing under your clothes can be a real turn-on for both the person who is wearing it as well as the person who is seeing it. After you've spent a long time selecting the perfect bra and panty set, why not let him savor it for a while? If you love the way her satin teddy feels against your skin, ask her to keep it on. Stockings can feel sexy as you rub your bodies together. And it's a turn on for women to feel a guy get hard through his underwear. Vivid director Justin Sterling is a fan of the partially dressed effect. "Sometimes I find it sexy to leave some clothes on," he says. "Sometimes I like the bra still on, or the panties. Sometimes it's nice and raw to just pull them aside. Clothes on are definitely sexy."

Vivid Girl Briana likes the undressing part to go very slow: "If the guy starts taking your clothes off too soon, just kind of coach him along. Most guys . . . know that you shouldn't just go in for the kill. If you tell them to slow down, hopefully they get the hint and will back up." No need to rush this part, since after all, it's erotic to have your lover unpeel your clothes and search for the parts of you they want to see or touch or taste.

Perhaps you want to capture the frenetic passion between you, and during those times, clothes just seem to be in the way. "I get really excited, and then I just want to do it fast. So I tear my clothes off real fast, myself. I always take everything off," says Dasha. "I like to strip the clothes off him. I like to pull his pants halfway down, and I usually leave them halfway down. It creates the feeling that you are so hot for each other, you can't wait until you're both naked." There is something hot about not removing one's clothes completely. Just push his pants down to his knees or pull up her dress. Of course, it depends upon the mood and how the passion is flowing. When the right moment comes, sometimes it feels right to just rip your clothes off as quickly as possible.

Sexy Clothes

❝❝ A lot of the guys in porn are turned on by shoes. I find that a lot of times leaving the shoes on during sex makes the girl's legs look really yummy. If I'm doing a spontaneous sex scene in a bathroom or alley, you never get totally nude. I like to keep some clothes on, a nice jock strap or tighty whiteys on the guy. ❞❞

—*Chi Chi LaRue, Vivid director*

Hands down, the women's clothing item sexiest to most guys is high-heeled boots and shoes. In porn films, you'll notice that the girls wear them in almost every scene, even in bed. Lots of guys like the black leather "biker chick" look, but there are others who find plain white pumps a turn-on. Whether platform heels or a tastefully pointed pair of pumps, the right shoes can be very enticing. Some psychologists theorize that our modern obsession with shoes as a sexy thing goes back to Victorian times when, because of long skirts and petticoats, a woman's ankle might be the only part of her you could see below the neck! Whatever the reason, both men and women are turned on by sexy shoes. So if you're a woman who enjoys wearing sexy stilettos, and your man is into it, try leaving them on in bed. Just for the record, the higher and tighter the boots, the sexier they are.

Where the Boys Aren't 14, where the action takes place in a tough, all-girl leather bar, is one of the best movies for sexy clothing. Thigh-high red or black patent-leather platform boots, leather collars with studs, suede chaps over thongs, tight ripped T-shirts and biker hats with chains are just a few of the erotic ensembles. Even the male go-go boys in the background are stripped down to their jocks. There's some sexy-kinky clothing in the same tough-girl genre in *Jenna Loves Rocco,* where one of the girls wears a bra made out of chains and shiny black leather. *Blondage* also features shiny thigh-high boots, studded bustiers, and leather strap-and-snap bras and thongs.

For those who like their sexy clothes on the softer side, there's a great pink lace corset, garter belt, and cutoff glove combination featured in *Savanna Superstar.* And if your style is more denim than lace, take a look at the really high cutoffs in *Where the Boys Aren't 15.* If you don't think you can carry off these types of things, wear some great lingerie that feels sensual and looks slinky. And don't overlook thigh-high stockings worn without panties—even under a business suit.

Women like to see guys looking sexy as well. Gone are the days when the stereotypical male porn star wore nothing more than a pair of black socks. Again, a partially clothed guy is somehow sexier than one who is completely nude. But that doesn't mean that all women are turned on by fancy silk boxers or skimpy Europeans bikinis. Most women would rather see a guy looking like himself, only with fewer clothes on. Depending on how often a guy's been to the gym, a good look might be bare-chested, with clingy track pants or pajama bottoms and nothing underneath. Or try the reverse under the covers by wearing a T-shirt and nothing else. Men should take a look at what the guys in the Vivid productions are or aren't wearing. For example, the football players wearing just their jerseys, socks, and cleats in *Student Body* look really hot. And the two samurai guys in *Lotus* do, too. Their erect penises peeking out of their partially open kimonos and, later, during a threesome when they are all bare except for their boots, make for some sexy visuals.

VIVID GIRL★ FAVORITES:

TIPS ON DRESSING AND CLOTHING

Mercedez: "We dress up at home. I dress up in my dance clothes, leave my heels on, and the table dance turns into sex."

Kira: "I love dressing up and corsets. I can't go out of the house without heels, and I run around the house in lingerie. Every man loves heels. I keep my heels on to have sex. They make your legs look sexy and, like lingerie, they make you feel sexy."

Sunrise: "For Christmas, I dressed up as a naughty elf, and my guy wore Santa Claus shorts."

Savanna: "Thigh-highs and garters are difficult to wear because they sometimes show through. But if I'm wearing a Chanel suit, I'll do it because it's easily camouflaged. And shoes are very important. I like to wear the highest shoes and keep them on later in the evening."

Jenna: "Guys hate lots of lipstick, especially lots of lip gloss; it's so sticky and so gross!"

Flirting

Whether you are meeting someone for the first time, or if you've been with them for ten years, flirting is one of those things that can spark romance and excitement between two people. For some people, sexual attraction can be an immediate, visceral experience. Kira, for example, says she likes people who are secure with themselves. For her, self-confidence is the biggest turn-on. "Lots of people play mind games," she says. "Some girls might say 'he's cute' or whatever, but 'he's hot' never goes through my head; it doesn't even register for me. When I start talking to a person, there's either chemistry or there's not."

Others, like Dasha, talk about reading signals and picking up on cues. "When you go into a bar as a woman, you see a man, he looks at you, you look a little bit later, and he looks again. If you like the look of the guy, then you give a little smile. The guy smiles back, and maybe orders a drink or sends a kiss through the air. There are many ways to do it. If she doesn't return your look or smile, then she's probably not open to that flirting thing. Make sure you get the first contact, eye contact. If it works, go on to the next step. Maybe send a note with the bartender. But make sure she returns your look so you don't end up feeling foolish." Dasha suggests that all women can tell the difference between a guy who is flirting because he's attracted, and one who is just out to score the next babe. "You totally can tell those guys who have studied pickup lines in magazines," she says. "You know, the guy can be sweet, but if you feel like he has studied for it, it just doesn't work. You want to say, 'Oh man, go do something else.' It just doesn't work. If the guy is natural, then you get the feeling this guy is okay."

Seduction

Everyone has their own erotic fantasies. Mercedez loves the fantasy of an exotic lover on a secluded island. "It's something I've never done, but who knows, maybe I'll get to film a scene like that in a movie. I've seen movies shot in tropical locations and they look like so much fun. It would be a very safe way to fulfill my fantasy." Another way, of course, is not to leave the bedroom at all, but to create the island in your mind.

Fantasies can bring you closer together and give you insight into each other. Bringing your fantasies to life can be a way to explore a different side of yourself or a new dynamic between the two of you. You can try something new, spice up your routine, or take your sexual relationship to the next level.

Whatever your scenario, whether you are dreaming of exotic locales or just anticipating a fun night with your lover, seduction is all about creating the right mood and connecting with your partner. Take your time, savor each moment, and it will enhance all the action that comes later. For some people, women especially, foreplay is the best part, and the slower it goes, the hotter the fire burns. Men, too, can benefit from a gradual buildup.

❝ ❝ I love being stroked and petted, when my partner runs his fingertips all over me, getting to know me and my body. I just love being caressed. That's not something we get to do in the movies much, but it's great at home. ❞ ❞

—*Sunrise*

If you have been with the same partner for a long time, expending energy on small physical things—like setting a sexy mood, flirting, and seducing your lover—can really add a new dimension to a monotonous routine. If you are relatively new to each other, taking small steps at first can help you to get to know your partner's body and their unique hot spots.

Vivid Girl Savanna Samson says, "I'm very touchy. I love to touch people, flirt, seduce. It can get me in trouble because sometimes people read it the wrong way and I don't even realize I'm doing it. When I want somebody, I will just do it. I'll run my fingers up my legs, run them through my hair. I love to whisper in ears and say nasty and tender things like 'You smell so good' and 'I can't tell you what I'm going to do for you later' and 'Let's get out of here!'" Savanna demonstrates two important tools of seduction, one verbal and one physical. Talking is a great way to break the ice, plus it can begin anywhere at any time—over dinner, at a party, or anytime throughout a date.

After talking comes touching. Holding hands, gentle caresses, and sensuous strokes will make your partner crave more. To really be able to get into sex, both of you need to be somewhat relaxed, with your minds and bodies on autopilot. A head massage is a great way to start. Some gentle pressure on the temples with the pads of your fingers moving in a circle can also relieve tension and feel really good. Then run your fingers or fingernails lightly through your partner's hair. Just the gentle stroking on their scalp will feel great.

Try giving each other sensual body massages. Use your thumbs to gently rub your partner's neck, shoulders, and upper back. Move along your partner's body gently and sensually, and talk to each other. This will open the channels of communication that will serve you well during more intimate activities later. If the upper-back rub is going well, move down to the lower back. If he or she is really enjoying it, keep it up and massage their rear end! And don't feel restricted to using your hands. Feathers, combs, necklaces, and even artist's paintbrushes can provide interesting sensations. It all depends on how you use them and on which part of the body. When your partner is ready to turn over or move on to something else, they'll let you know. Foreplay is critical for Briana, who says, "I like a lot of kissing, a lot of foreplay. I like getting the back of my neck rubbed, and him touching me on the outside of my clothes before he starts going under my clothes. I like to be made to want it."

Justin suggests either the head or the feet as a good place to start. "If a girl is lying back on you, give her a head message. Kiss [her] on the neck, maybe let her suck on your finger and then get a kiss. The feet are a good choice—not too difficult, and very sensitive for some women," he says. Dasha adds, "What gets me is when a guy goes for my neck. My neck is so sensitive; go and lick it a little bit and rub it, go a little on my ear, and I'm ready to go." For Sunrise, the eyes have it. "I think the thing I like doing most is looking into my lover's eyes. I love to get to know people by staring in their eyes and trying to see through them, to see what is making them do the things they do, what drives them. It's amazingly good foreplay."

Slow dancing, like massage, is another great excuse to touch each other. Put on some soft music and invite your partner to join you. Just hold each other and rock from side to side. No style or fancy steps are needed! Look into each other's eyes from time to time, and put your head on your partner's shoulder, or bury your nose in their hair.

❝ ❝ I love a really slow buildup; the
slower he goes, the better. I could
probably come in five minutes, but if
a guy is skilled in the art of teasing,
then I can be teased for a half hour
or forty-five minutes, that's really
intense. ❞ ❞

—Jenna Jameson

Watching an adult video or DVD with your partner is another way to get the ball rolling. But you also might take some time to watch a few by yourself to see how the pros do it. One simple way to begin is in the shower or bath, and *Bangkok Nights* shows a sailor's seduction with a soapy bath sponge.

Savanna uses her experience in strip clubs to make foreplay its own show. "I like him to strip down," she says. "I don't like fumbling with buttons. But I do like to undress myself slowly and have him watch me as I'm doing it; sometimes with a little skirt. I used to be a dancer, and I'll do a little dance, slowly take the dress off." Even if you've never been a stripper, you can still give your partner a great striptease. The key is removing your clothing gradually, and not allowing him to touch you while you are teasing and revealing what is underneath. There's an interesting strip show in *Jenna Loves Rocco,* and another slow, sensual sort of striptease given by a woman in a bedroom window in *Looking In.* For cues on lap dancing, turn on *I Married a Porn Star,* or take a peek at *Blondage* for some serious hair tossing, pole licking, and grinding your body to music.

If you like things a little rougher, *Domination Nation* has an exciting scene that includes stretching a pair of panties really tight and rubbing them back and forth over a woman's clit area. Or take a look at the scene in *Where the Boys Aren't 14,* where Dasha massages another woman's pussy with the toe of her boot, then rips open her panties with the sharp stiletto heel.

Communication: Telling Someone What You Want

Before we get into some physical techniques you can put into practice, it's important for you to explore your desires and learn to communicate them to your partner. Remember, you are the director of this erotic production. You know the characters, and you know where you want the story to go. Sharing what you need, what you want, and what your fantasies are will create a fulfilling experience for both of you. Talking to each other builds intimacy and increases the connection between you. What you say to each other before you get down and dirty can be a crucial part of seduction and foreplay.

It seems strange that people who are having sex together might find it difficult to talk to each other about what they want. They might be inhibited about suggesting something new or afraid of sounding too weird. They might worry that they will "kill the moment" if they say the wrong thing. Or they may be afraid that if they say what they want ("Harder! Right there! Up a little!"), their partner might feel criticized or inadequate. Mercedez admits, "Talking during sex embarrasses me—I don't want to answer fifty questions! I'm more into sounds, like moaning, than actually talking. Sounds are sexy, and they can also say just as much as words." The first thing to remember is that the best sex comes with a partner who is open to suggestions, and who is more concerned with your needs than with his or her own image of themselves as a perfect lover. Second, even a perfect lover needs some coaching from time to time as they get to know your body and your needs. Sure, it's great when no words are necessary, and you just seem to be reading each other's mind, but sometimes a little verbal coaching can help.

On the other hand, sometimes you don't want or need to be too specific. You may be afraid to break the mood, or not sure of what your partner's reaction would be. There is nothing wrong with dropping hints. If you really want him to slip his hands into your panties, pushing his hand in that direction will probably give him the idea. But if you aren't sure of your partner's nonverbal cues, or are new to each other, you definitely need to open your mouth. To get what you want in bed, some negotiation is almost always necessary.

When love and sex are concerned, it's crucial to realize that you are the best source of information about your sexuality—you know what turns you on and gets you off. So you need to find the courage and confidence to say it out loud. Don't be afraid to play director, and give someone clear instructions about what you like, such as how slow or fast, how soft or hard, how deep, or, well, you get the idea. As Sunrise says, "I love someone to tell me what they like and what turns them on. I love to be guided. It reassures me that I am doing a good job!" Savanna concurs: "Even though I am supposed to know what I am doing, everyone is so different. So it's great when people give me direction, tell me what they want!"

If you've been with your partner for a while, try talking about what you want before you're in the middle of the action. When shooting a film, the director usually tells the actors what he or she wants before they begin shooting a scene. Maybe there's a little fine tuning between takes, such as "Move your leg a little more to the left next time." But there are usually no stage directions given while the camera is rolling. Similarly, the best time for you and your partner to talk about what you like is before sex—not during. It's not a great idea to talk about this right after sex because it may sound as though you're critiquing your partner's performance.

Do you want her to wear something scandalous? Do you wish your partner had a softer and more sensual touch, or one that was harder, tighter, and more energetic? Do you want oral sex to last longer? If you want to introduce something new into your bedroom routine, like a position you've never tried or a sex toy, and you're not sure how your partner will react, then pitching the idea during sex may put the brakes on. So introduce the idea at a more neutral time and place. Kira says, "The best thing you can do is ask your partner what he wants. Ask, 'Does this feel good? What's your favorite thing, what's something you want to try?' I know what it's like to be afraid to say that, but it works." New adventures should always be up for discussion: talk about why you'd like to do something, what about it turns you on, and how you envision it happening. Get feedback and input from your partner.

The purpose of talking it over is to try to bring your expectations and your partner's together. If you are expecting a slow, gentle, romantic night, and she's geared up for a quickie on the kitchen table, you could both end up disappointed. If one partner is unsure of something, try a compromise where they can agree to dip a toe in the water rather then plunging headlong into the pool. Keep listening to each other. And after you try anything new, talk about what happened and whether you'll go further next time, or pull back. Kira says, "How you bring something up depends on the person. If your partner is more conservative, you could be indirect, and say, 'A friend of mine is into this, what do you think?' I think lots of men are really open to new things, you just have to speak up."

Sometimes you feel an urgent need to tell your partner what you want, where you want it, and how you like it at that very moment. "I just come right out and tell him exactly what I want him to do," says Sunrise. "There is nothing wrong with saying what you want. When I am in the right mood, I can really take control and direct my partner, be really verbal. I tell them what to do and how to do it. It is such a turn-on." One terrific tease is to direct your partner to masturbate. Tell him he only gets to stroke himself ten times and then he has to stop. Or she has to put on a show for you, following all your instructions to the letter.

What you say during sex can engage your mind and imagination to enhance the sensations your body experiences. There are many ways to converse during a scene. Your words can range from normal conversation to sweet nothings, from hints about what you want to really raunchy, raw talk. You may discover that a minimum of talking is best for you, or you may open up entirely new erotic possibilities for yourself and your partner. Talking during sex can be, as Vivid director Chi Chi LaRue puts it, "a real turn-on and a stimulator. When performers talk to each other or even whisper kind of nasty things, they both get turned on, and the scene immediately becomes more intense."

The Vivid performers are used to communicating about sex. When a performer works with someone new, they must quickly let their partner know their likes and dislikes. You, however, may be a little more shy. So try this: practice saying what you want out loud when you are by yourself—like an actor reciting your lines. The more at ease you become with speaking the words, the more comfortable you'll be with doing the deed. Before you dish out orders (diplomatically!) to your costar, it's a good idea to begin with a compliment, as in, "That feels really good, and I would love it if you'd . . ." Or, as Savanna says, "It's better to say what you like to your partner rather than what you don't like." Your direction should be gently delivered but absolutely explicit—this is no time to be vague! Dasha recommends directness: "I just tell guys what I want straight out. Why make it difficult? I'm not going to do something like push him in that general direction and hope he gets the idea— if you do that, you'll just end up disappointed. He cannot read your mind."

❝❝ **Communication is the most important part of a relationship; don't hesitate to tell your partner about your fantasies. In my experience, the more open I am, the more receptive my partner is.** ❞❞

—*Savanna*

Communication is also critical when it comes to conveying your fantasies. Maybe you want to try something special with a lover you've known for a long time. Maybe there's something you've never done, or something you've been waiting to do. Have you fantasized about role-playing? Imagined having sex in a different location? Is there a fantasy you have or an idea you'd like to try that you read about in a book or saw in a movie? Watch that movie together, or share the book with him or her. Give your partner a chance to get used to the idea, and listen to their reaction. If they sound interested, you can talk more about whether you are going to try it.

❝❝ **Guys, if you feel like doing something, don't be scared, just ask your girl. You want to be with a person who is open-minded, someone who wants to please you and won't turn her nose up at a new suggestion. If she's open to things, you'll see that you mean something to her.** ❞❞

—*Dasha*

If you are watching a movie, gauge your partner's reaction and be honest about how you feel. Or how about writing your fantasy in a love letter? Sometimes it's easier to say it on paper than directly to your lover's face. Use some nice stationery to make the idea inviting and romantic, no matter how raunchy it may be! Or send a sexy e-mail.

Kira warns against pressuring your partner: "I think the worst feeling is when you feel like your partner is judging you if you don't embrace their idea immediately. If you don't push me, I feel like I can take an idea and sit with it for a while, and come to it at my own pace." Therefore, it might be best to "float" your idea a few times and see what the reaction is; a lot of people need time to think about something. But you should never feel pressured, or pressure your partner about doing something.

> ❛❛ **If your partner is trying to pressure you into something, it's going to scare you more. You'll put it in your head that you have to do it for them. You have to be sure that you're ready, you're with a person you trust, and it's the right time . . . You can feel violated if you do something you didn't really want to. If you are going to do anything, you have to do it for YOU. Whatever it is, when the time comes, to let someone in like that, can be very special and sacred.** ❜❜
>
> —*Sunrise*

3
lip service

Fantasy File:

She trembles slightly as she is led into the royal bed-chamber by the cunning man who serves as chief adviser to the Emperor. As one of the many court concubines, she knows what fate awaits her if her plan fails. She has watched the process happen for many days now. One by one, beautiful concubines were brought before the powerful ruler to fill his bed and his lustful appetite, yet none had ever returned. On the advice of the Emperor's adviser, it was decreed that every woman who had lain with the Emperor would be put to death the next morning so that no other man would have her.

The exquisite girl feels her nipples becoming firm as they rub against the silk of her embroidered kimono. Taking tiny steps, she bows as she enters the bedchamber. When she lifts her eyes, she sees the Emperor in all his splendor. Beneath his blue-and-gold robe, he possesses a magnificent body along with the fine-looking features on his regal face. "You will have to wait," he tells her, grimacing and glancing down beneath his robe. "That is all right, Your Excellency," she answers. "I have one hundred ways to get you hard without even touching you." "How can that be?" he asks. "One hundred and one, actually," she answers respectfully.

"Let me tell you the story about the stable boy," she begins. "Although he was very fair to look at, his brain was a little off, as he was very much in love with the lady of the manor." Intrigued, the Emperor claps his hands twice, signaling his adviser to leave and bolt the doors behind him so they are alone. "Do continue," he commands.

"The lady of the manor lusted for the stable boy, but she knew the lust could never see the light of day, and she knew what went on behind closed doors." As the charming concubine continues her narration, the Emperor can almost hear the wind chimes as she describes every detail of the scene. And he feels himself hardening as he watches her luscious mouth form the words of her story. She tells him how the beautiful lady sits fanning herself as she and her white parrot are carried around in a rattan rickshaw by the stable boy.

"The stable boy had the chiseled muscles and hard body of a fine youth," the concubine continues, "and in the hot sun, he wore only his chest plate, armbands, and peasant trousers. When he put down the rickshaw to rest for a moment, the lady watched him wash his broad chest and muscular arms with cool water from the trough. When the boy asked if the lady was ready to continue their journey, she demurely asked him to remove her shoes and massage her feet, as they were hot and tired from the journey. Then, after instructing the stable boy to remove all but his trousers, the lady placed her tiny foot against the boy's massive, sweating chest, and slowly ran her toes down to the folds that covered his manhood. They looked into each other's eyes with overwhelming love and desire, and the two rapidly removed the rest of their clothing and stood naked in the hot afternoon sun. Her tiny frame leaned against his powerful body as she caressed his face. They kissed tenderly. With one strong hand he embraced her, feeling the softness of her breasts against his arm. And with the other, he delicately massaged her growing clit as she moaned with lust. He laid her back against the rickshaw and, with a skill beyond his age, massaged her wanting clit and pussy with his broad wet tongue. When the lady was thoroughly satisfied, she dropped down to the ground to demonstrate her respect for this gentle, beautiful boy, and took his enormous, turgid member in her mouth. The boy cried out with pleasure as she wrapped her hands around him, sucking and licking every inch. Then, when it was time, he swooped her up in his arms, and with one deft move, placed her ankles on his shoulders and began his ferocious thrusting inside her. Tiring, they switched positions so that her delicate belly leaned over the side of the rickshaw, and he could take her fiercely like a mongrel dog. When the time had come for him to end, she presented him with her shoe as a vessel that would forever contain the living liquid of their pleasures. She held him tightly as the white, milky fluid reached its target. And after he had spurt the last of his man juice, she placed her foot inside the shoe that would hold their secret forever."

"That was a strong recollection," says the Emperor, "almost as though you had been there yourself." She smiles as she slides effortlessly onto the bed, and allows her kimono to fall open, revealing her succulent body. Looking resplendent on the jewel-colored satin sheets amid the tower of pillows, the concubine begins to tug and twist on her tiny pink nipples as the Emperor watches eagerly. "But you told me there were one hundred different ways," the Emperor questions. "One hundred and one, O Radiant One," answers the girl. "Indulge me," he says with pleasure. "Of course, Your Excellency," she says with a modest smile, "but that is another story."

★★ *from* Lotus, *directed by*
Ralph Parfait

Romance

66 **Sex is a powerful force and one of the most exciting things about it is that it can be very spontaneous. You can expand your horizons; trips into unexplored territory can fuel a wonderful relationship.** 99

—*Vivid director Paul Thomas*

Even the irrepressible Vivid Girls have their special, private desires and sexual fantasies. The difference between the Vivid Girls and many people, though, is that these women have no qualms about filling their bedroom with flowers, lighting candles or incense, putting satin sheets on the bed, and making themselves up beautifully, and *then* doing what comes naturally when that special man gets home. Through their line of work, the women of Vivid have found that place in themselves where they can grab a sexual fantasy and make it reality without shame, hesitation, or guilt. Our goal is to get you to that same place.

66 **For me, romance is when it's all about us; the focus is on an erotic evening.** 99

—*Savanna*

When we think of romance, we usually think of something sentimental, emotional, or full of passion and desire. Romance is something extraordinary—a wonderful, fanciful idea that appeals to everyone. In the tale of the Emperor and the concubine, romance flourishes when a very special woman does what no other had been able to do before—excite the Emperor's imagination and arouse his physical senses without even touching him. The concubine is so fascinating to the Emperor because she does something unique, and her allure is that she had planned her seduction specifically for him. Not everyone is gifted at telling stories like Scheherazade, or the concubine in our story, but we are all capable of being romantic. Romance often involves doing something for another person that is out of the ordinary, and that displays or expresses our love and desire for them.

66 **What is romantic? For me it's typical; a nice dinner, rose petals on the bed . . . making the night unique.** 99

—*Tawny*

Everyone has a different idea of what is romantic. According to Jenna, "Anything you do to change your environment and make it seem special is going to add to the evening." On Valentine's Day, for example, many people rely on the usual tokens of affection—roses, chocolates, cute stuffed animals, sexy lingerie, a pair of silk boxers, or dinner at a romantic restaurant. But if you want to make sex romantic, sometimes you have to move beyond the basics.

66 **I like to pick out a really sexy outfit, and select one for my partner, then we give each other a personal fashion show. I like all kinds of sexy clothes—nighties, teddies, stockings, stilettos.** 99

—*Sunrise*

Usually, when a guy goes over to a woman's place with sex in mind, he focuses on the woman and not on the surroundings. But most women are a little bit different—they take it all in. Justin offers some advice for guys about how to prep your place for a night of sex. "I'm re-

★VIVID GIRL★ FAVORITES:

ally into lighting for creating the mood . . . lights dimmed down low, candles. Trying to push it with music can be too much, [so] turn MTV down low. Have some chilled wineglasses, and a glass of wine at the ready." He also suggests turning down the bed in advance and, maybe, having some sex toys readily at hand. But his advice also goes beyond the basics to things that most women will notice and really appreciate. "If it's a first-time date," says Justin, "make sure your place is clean, ready, and guys, make sure that your towels are clean and there's toilet paper. Clean your kitchen, put fresh sheets on your bed, and have some respect for yourself. I think how you keep your house is a direct sign of how you respect yourself and how you respect others in your relationship—even if you have to hide everything under the bed."

After you set the stage for romance and seduction, you're ready to begin. "I like when a guy starts out slow, and I'm not sure exactly what he's going to do next.

Whatever he does is a surprise—that drives me crazy," says Briana. Kira agrees. "I like men who are about pleasing their partners and taking their time."

Kissing Like a Pro

❝ **Kissing has to be one of the most important things when it comes to sex. I think men need to learn to take it slow. Instead of just diving right in and trying to engulf my whole face, just keep it really soft. Focus on me, and you'll really get this girl's blood pressure going.** ❞

—Jenna

Kisses are one of the first intimate actions lovers share. On a first date, that good-night kiss at the door may be what determines whether or not you dream of each other until the next date. Depending on your style and delivery, a kiss can express many emotions: love, passion, desire, affection, or domination, to name a few. There are many kinds of kisses and many of us are very finicky about how we like them—soft, hard, wet, or dry. In fact, the Vivid film *The Kiss* is a tongue-in-cheek sex comedy that's all about kissing. In the film, a girl seems to have the perfect boyfriend—good-looking, sexy and rich; but she's not happy. Why? Because her boyfriend is a lousy kisser. Meanwhile, her male roommate has a secret crush on her, and boasts to his friend that he can make her fall for him if he just gets a chance to kiss her. The rest of the film presents some hilarious, ill-fated strategies for making that happen. *Never* underestimate the power of a kiss!

What's right for a first kiss might be too light when in the throes of passion; likewise, a really sloppy face plant can be overwhelming if given too early in the evening. Like many things sensual, you need to read your partner's reactions and respond to each other's preferences. But kissing is a way to quickly heat things up for both of you. In fact, it's been said that any lover who can master the art of the kiss is more than halfway to greatness.

> ❝ **The most important moment in the evening would have to be the first kiss. A great first kiss takes your breath away and gives you butterflies in your stomach.** ❞
>
> —*Jenna*

A first kiss can be like a first impression; it sets the tone for the rest of the evening and leaves a lasting mark. "The first kiss should be very light, almost a tease," says Justin. "You have to extract the desire from them—maybe then just a touch with the tongue and kiss her neck." Overall, the women in our crew preferred firm lips, but a soft and light kiss. "I like soft lips," says Mercedez, "no slobbering!" And most of them admired the way one of the actors, Rocco Siffredi, engages in tender before-and-after kissing and cuddling on screen. To take a look at Rocco's style close up, check out the film *Chasey Loves Rocco*. Another suggestion is *Good Time Girl,* which has some great kissing scenes as well.

You might want to start with this tease of a kiss. Lean forward as though you are going to kiss. Open your mouth slightly. But as your two mouths near, move your head slightly to one side so that your lips just barely brush, or perhaps miss completely. You can move it to the other side on the same pass, and underscore the moment with the soft brush on the lips with clean, lightly scented hair. Or, as you bring your lips together, nibble gently at the edges of your partner's mouth (using your lips, not your teeth). He or she may nibble back, or if that's a bit of a tease for them, may grab you and do something way more passionate back!

Mercedez equates the kiss with being teased: "I only like the kissing near the beginning. I don't like to be kissed too much; it's just a prelude to other things for me. I know some women you could just kiss all night, but for me, kiss me just enough to tease me. I think the lips are the sexiest part of a man. I like looking at his lips." Tawny is the opposite: "It depends on how horny I am, but there are times when I definitely like a lot of kissing. I like to just get lost in his arms."

Men: let your mouths come together softly when you plant one on her, then move them against each other with small movements of your lips and head. Remember Justin's suggestion to "extract the desire" from her. That means always go softer than you think you should. If she wants it harder, she'll kiss back harder or grab you harder. Tawny says: "Some guys are too aggressive. I don't like it when someone shoves their tongue down my throat. I prefer gentle kisses." Some people like to let the very tip of their tongue slip between their lips for a moment—just enough for your partner to feel it. It can be a tasty tease, and also a good way to wet your lips just a little, so you can prolong the kiss. You can do it several times in quick succession. If your partner starts to breathe faster or harder, it's working. On the other hand, some people want to get on with more luscious lip action. Try using your tongue to lightly trace an outline over your partner's lips. This works as a really good tease—as long as it's not like a big sloppy wet one from the family dog. Another Vivid Girl tip: don't even think about making smoochy, smacker noises during a sexy kiss. That kind of kissing sound should be reserved for throwing kisses in the direction of puppies and kittens, or for when you're on the telephone and the other person can hear you but not feel you.

Most people close their eyes reflexively when they kiss. It's nice to get caught up in the moment, and lose yourself in a deep, passionate smooch. You surrender to your partner, and let your mouths and bodies meld. But sometimes it can be incredibly hot to make eye contact while you kiss. It allows you to read the emotions and feelings of your partner. Experiment to see what feels comfortable for you.

6 6 Kiss her all over—her ears, her neck . . . but don't slobber all over the place, and not too much tongue. 9 9

—*Jenna*

Everyone agrees that using your tongue is a plus, as long as you don't go overboard and get sloppy. Sunrise says she hates when a guy engulfs her mouth completely. "The mouth has to be a little bit firm and not too much saliva," cautions Dasha. "The right kiss just does it. If it is too messy it's a turnoff." The classic French kiss involves both of your tongues. The goal here for the guys is not to ram his tongue down her throat, but to get your two tongues together. The tongue is very sensitive and the sensation of something teasing it can be quite pleasurable. Savanna offers some very clear specs for her ideal kiss: "I like the lips to touch and then the tongue to go in; then tongue on tongue. I don't like wide-open kisses and I don't like small mouth kisses. I don't like it with too much saliva—just some lip and then soft tongue, not a hard tongue."

One fun trick to do with the tongue is to pull your partner's tongue into your mouth. It usually starts the other way around, with your tongue in your partner's mouth. As you pull it back into your own mouth, if your lips are close together and airtight, their tongue will be "sucked" right in. You may have to suck gently to create the airtight seal in the first place, but don't suck too hard. You'll take his or her breath away with this move as it is. Another variation on the French kiss is to trace the surface of your partner's lower and upper teeth with your tongue. And remember her other parts, too (which we'll explore soon). To check out some really long, deep kisses, note the final scenes between the Emperor and the concubine in *Lotus*, where she starts kissing up on top and works her way down. "Kissing on the neck, behind the ear, and on the belly," says Briana, "those are also very important spots for me."

While your mouths are busy, other parts of you can be active as well. Stroke each other's back, hair, cheeks. Many women especially respond to caresses on the neck. Remember to touch very lightly with your fingers. You can also run your fingers through her hair, and even give a little tug. "Hair is a very important thing to remember and manage correctly while you're kissing," says Justin. "You have to know how to pull on a girl's hair. It's a little bit of a dominating thing. But girls with really tender scalps don't like it. You have to learn how to run your hand up her neck and into her hair, then just tighten a little bit—don't yank a chunk out!" If you're both standing up when you do this, you have to be taller than she is for it to work. Otherwise you'll tip her lips up and away from you. If she's taller, or in very tall heels, you might want to stand behind her while she's sitting, or lie down first. For women who really love the hands-on-the-hair move, it can make their knees go weak, so have a bed or couch handy to collapse onto, or be prepared to hold her up with your other arm. If she has a really tender head, you'll hear "ouch!" (or something more graphic) instead of "aaaah," and you'll know she's not into it.

Sunrise says, "I like really deep and passionate kisses. When someone kisses me, I really want to feel the passion." Speaking of moving beyond soft and sweet, Kira offers, "When you're really into it, you want that really hard kiss, especially if you're doing rough sex. You can always play down and do the sensual stuff later." A hard, fast, or slightly forceful kiss should be delivered when the mood is right. Work your way up to it, and at the appropriate moment, kick it up a notch. Kira sums up the significance of a strong lip-lock: "Kisses can be more intense than anything else. You never know what you are going to get, but if the chemistry is there, you connect and it works."

More Pleasure Spots to Explore

"" I call my neck and ears 'the forbidden zones,' because when you lick them, I go crazy! I also like my lower back kissed. When someone did it for the first time, it drove me insane, even more than my neck and ears. ""

—*Kira*

We wouldn't be doing you, or your partner, justice, if we didn't mention some "out of the way" places you might want to explore with your lips. As Vivid actor Bobby Vitale puts it, "The more spots you touch the more pleasure it gives her. Rub on her face gently; gently go around her lips, slide your hands down her throat, and then grab her by the chin to let her feel how passionate you are." Many of these spots are great to try on men, too.

Different parts of the neck are sensitive depending on the person. For some, the area behind the ear, or just below it, is the most sensitive. For others, the magic spot is closer to the collarbone, while still more have it on the back of their neck, just below their hairline. Explore these places with your tongue, all the while reading your lover's reaction. When you hit a spot they especially like, stick with it for a while, lick it and nibble it, and then come back to that area again as the night goes on. As your partner becomes more aroused, that place may become even more sensitive. Just be sure that all your ear and neck licking doesn't send your partner into fits of laughter; they might be ticklish. "I think men just like attention, period," muses Jenna. "When women take their time and go over their whole body, their whole body is an erogenous zone. I've noticed that men really, really like it when girls kiss their neck, though." You don't have to lick or nibble very long before you give your lover electric shivers all up and down his or her body! And then some gentle suction will heighten the sensation. Just be careful of sucking and biting, unless you are both prepared for a visible mark.

Ears are another very hot spot for many of the Vivid girls. Savanna says, "I go crazy when someone kisses my neck and my ears." For many women and men, the ears are a surefire way to send the blood rushing to all the right places. Try licking the outside of the ear; tracing the grooves and ridges with your tongue. While there, you may also want to whisper a few choice things. Nibble or suck on the earlobes, kiss the back of the ears, and see how your partner responds. If they say "ugh" or "cut it out," just move on to somewhere else on their body.

Another favorite spot of Savanna's is "that muscle that goes from the hip bone down to the groin on either side of a man." Use the flat part of your tongue or nibble him (or her) on the hip, and in the crease between the leg and the torso. There are many nerve endings here that are near the nerves of the sex organs. Stimulating along these areas can spill over into stimulating the entire region. Jenna loves this area on herself: "Right where your hip bone is, if a guy bites right there very softly . . ." On her partner, she likes to tease him a bit in the pelvic area. "I like kissing all around him, instead of just his dick, and it drives them crazy, like 'when is she going to put her mouth on me!'"

Dasha also likes the idea of teasing areas that are near the crucial ones: "A woman's belly is really sexy, and it's halfway between two important parts of her body." Use your tongue and lips to trace a line down the center of your partner's chest and stomach, down the sternum, and straight down from the belly button toward the "fun stuff" below. One of the important main nerves involved with orgasm, the vagus nerve, travels down everyone's front. The line from the belly button below can be especially electric to women who feel an "echo" of sensation there in their clits. Briana identifies her most sensitive spots as "my neck, around my belly button, and my inner thighs."

A good rule is that almost anywhere you can find a "valley" on the body, whether it's the crease between the leg and torso we talked about before, or places like the back of the knee or the crook of the elbow, you will find soft, sensitive flesh waiting to be stimulated. Bobby's favorite part of a woman is "in between her thighs, her pussy, and her ass, I call it the peach. There's a little gap there. It's a nice sweet spot and you need to be able to get right down there to taste it."

Fingers are remarkably erotic parts of the body, and using them in different ways and in different places can deliver great results. Experiment with light tapping, stroking up and down, or in a circle. Using one finger or several fingers will provide different sensations, as will gently pinching and rolling a small bit of flesh between your thumb and forefinger. And don't forget about seductively putting your fingers in your partner's mouth. You can see some good examples of finger licking in *The Vision*. Other examples of this and putting your fingers in your partner's mouth—or putting *their* fingers in *your* mouth—are in *Swoosh*.

Don't forget the back of the body as well. Kira's keen on her backside: "One place we just discovered was my lower back. He did some really light kissing and I was like 'whoa, that's really got me!'" Savanna and Jenna have a similar weakness: their knees. Jenna says, "I'd rather the man licked the back of my knees. That's something that really turns me on, places that are often ignored. The backs of my knees are really sensitive. When I'm getting a massage, I'll start to purr."

Tawny is gung ho for a good toe sucking, and she's not the only one. "I love my toes sucked," she says. "It feels really good. I have done it in private and on film, and it is an awesome feeling, one that's really different from anything else. Of course, I take a shower, get a pedicure, and make sure my feet and toes are smooth and ready for action." People also like to play with each other's body using their toes. An example of this is in the film *The Audition*, where the man's toe tickling goes straight for the clit. Another erotic move in that movie is watching yourselves in the mirror to get even more excited.

Everyone is unique, as are the erotic places they like to have touched and teased. Even among the Vivid Girls, erogenous zones vary greatly. It's important to explore each other's body and not rule out any part off the bat: you may find a sensitive spot where you least expect it.

Another Way to Use Your Mouth: Dirty Talk

" " I finally got into dirty talk! I prefer to listen and once in a while open my mouth, but if he's not saying anything, I will. It definitely makes sex hotter. " "

—Kira

Maybe you remember the scene in *Bangkok Nights* in which one of the brothel's regular clients asks his favorite prostitute to tell him, in great detail, about the sex she had with some of the other male visitors. Or the scene in *Intimate Journey* in which a woman describes her first experience with anal sex in painstaking detail. Dirty talk is sexy talk. And hearing it can often help conjure up the naughtiest fantasies in one's imagination. Dirty talk sounds really funny, or trashy, when you're not having sex. But within the right context—like, let's say, the throes of passion—it can be a major turn-on.

Where would adult movies be without the words "oh yeah, oh yeah"? Dialogue is actually a big part of porn. Chi Chi says, "I remember when videos just had music sound tracks back in the early 1980s. When the first movies [came] out with dialogue and dirty talk, it was just so thrilling and [it] added another level to the scenes. And talk is very safe. You can say a lot of nasty things that you'd never actually do." What you say during sex can connect your mind and imagination to enhance the sensations your body feels.

We all know that whether you're in the boardroom or the bedroom, sometimes it isn't what you say, but how you say it. There are many ways to converse during a scene; your words can range from normal conversation to sweet nothings, from hints about what you want to raunchy and raw talk. You may discover that a minimum of talking is best for you, or you might open up a whole new range of erotic possibilities. Talking during sex can be, as Chi Chi says, "a real turn-on and a stimulator. When performers talk to each other or even whisper kind of nasty things, they both get turned on, and the scene immediately becomes more intense." Kira said she even brought the dialogue from the set to her bedroom at home: "I had a boyfriend who kept doing it and it totally turned me off. But then with my next boyfriend, I felt something was missing, so I found myself talking, and now he's doing it, too. I prefer to listen, but once in a while I throw some words in for myself. If he's not saying anything, I will. It makes it hotter!"

Erotic talk can vary from mild to wild. What you say and how you say it depends on your style, your mood, and what's happening between the sheets. An easy way to begin sex talk is simply to verbalize how much you like your partner's looks, what your partner is doing, or how it makes you feel. Everyone likes to have their ego stroked as much as other parts of their body. Telling your partner how beautiful or handsome they are can build their confidence, and the more confident they are, the better they can please you, and the more they can enjoy themselves. Plus, they are less likely to stop what they are doing to you. So if you want them to keep it up, keep talking! Dasha, whose native language is Czech, says, "I have an easier time talking dirty in English than I do in Czech. I don't even know how to talk dirty in Czech because it sounds silly in that language. But in English, I hear people do it all the time and it's easier; it adds a little spice."

You can also narrate the action in a sexy way: talk about what you're doing to your partner, what your partner is doing to you, say what you want to do, or what you're going to do. This all seems pretty basic, but in an erotic context, it really can add something to the experience for both partners. Choosing the words depends on what feels right and how hot and heavy you are. If you want to open up the dialogue, but feel uncomfortable using street slang, say something relatively tame like "I'm going to make you scream tonight." If you haven't got a problem using slang, or lines you picked up in a movie, try something more explicit, such as "I'm going to give you the best blow job you ever had." This cranks things up a notch. And if and when you're fairly comfortable with talking dirty, you can progress to something like "I'm gonna suck your dick so hard and so long that you'll be begging me to let you come." See what we mean? The more explicit it is, the more exciting it can be; especially if you only use this sort of talk in the bedroom.

"I'm more of a sounds person; moans and things," says Mercedez. "Hearing sexy sounds can turn me on even more than hearing words. But sometimes, it helps to get him hard by telling dirty stories, or saying how bad I want it, or I tell him what I'm going to do when it gets hard. I tell him what kind of blow job I'm going to give him, and then I'll do it." Briana keeps it simple: "Whispering in your ear is a great kind of foreplay. In my scenes, I just say what comes naturally, like what I am going to do to my partner or what I want him to do to me. Once in a while raunchy is okay, but for the most part, I'm not into gutter talk; I keep it sweet and hot."

If you'd really like to see our Vivid actors using dirty talk so that you can decide if it's right for you, check out *The Most Beautiful Girl in the World*. The words seem out of context here, but when Tawny says to her boyfriend in the film, "Do you want to fuck me?" and "Faster, you fucking bitch; make me come," it seems perfectly right for the hard ass character she's playing. And remember, while you're having sex with someone, you can momentarily take on a different character as well. In *Swoosh,* a girl in the swimming-pool scene uses words that are hot but not vulgar when she says to a guy, "I'm nice and wet for you, huh?" But later in the same film, there's a scene in a remote shack that serves as a hideout for some tough-guy types and their babes. There, the talk is raunchier, with lines like "Is that what you want, you fuckin' filthy whore?" Or "Take it, bitch." Or "Fuck me with that stick, baby."

No one wants a one-way conversation. To inspire your other

half, ask questions like "How does this feel?" or "Do you like what I am doing?" Pay attention to your delivery because a little breathiness for women, and a little forcefulness for men, can go a long way. You don't want to sound too businesslike or neutral, like a masseuse in a health spa, or the nurse in a hospital who just changed the bed linens. Put a little edge in your voice.

A fun little bedroom game is to take turns asking for something special that you want. It can be a foot rub, a blow job, or a spanking. This can be a great tactic for extending foreplay, too, if it seems like your partner needs to slow down a bit. Bobby encourages versatility: "There is a wide range of things I can say, depending on the scene. One minute I can whisper 'you're the most beautiful thing on earth' and touch her face and kiss her. Then I can cover her eyes and tell her what a dirty girl she is. I can be romantic or I can be naughty. It's a balance. I make her desired, secure, and safe. Then I can push the envelope sexually with what I say."

When most people think of "talking dirty" they think of using nasty, even degrading, language to make it hot. When it works, it works well! Dirty talk can really supercharge the eroticism for those who get off on it, but we have a delicious paradox here. The dialogue in adult movies is not always brilliant, and if we're not aroused it can sound downright silly. But when we are aroused dirty talk can stoke the fires even hotter by engaging our minds as well as our bodies. The trick is to say the kinds of things you hear adult performers say, but not to sound like you're in a porn movie when you say it. "I don't like nasty talk, but I like sweet nasty talk," says Bobby. "Instead of hearing 'fuck my hole,' I would rather she said something ladylike, like 'give it to me harder, baby,' or I just like to hear her whimpers." Sunrise, for example, says she has no problem talking dirty on the set, but she doesn't really do it very much at home. "At work I'm a major talker, especially if I'm with a female. I can take control and give verbal commands and stuff like that. Say I'm holding her hair forcefully and telling her to 'eat me,' or 'fuck me with your tongue.' It's such a turn-on. And what you say doesn't even have to make sense for you to enjoy it!"

Remember, the goal in your scene is to have great sex with your partner—the only audience or director you have to please is you! "Me, myself, I'm not a big dirty talker," says Jenna. "I think it can be hot, but guys can go too far and say something that turns me off, then it throws my whole groove off. Maybe some things will come out of my mouth that a guy will really dig, but once you get going, it's important to concentrate on what you're doing. Moans and groans are hotter and more real for me." Generally speaking, you both have to be really into it for dirty talk to work. If one of you isn't into it, at best it will fall flat, and at worst you'll actually offend your partner. If there are certain words or phrases that bug you, by all means, let your partner know. Guys take careful note here; women are more sensitive than men to slang words that refer to breasts and vaginas. For some women, "boobs" are okay, but "hooters" is unacceptable. Similarly, some women will think that "snatch" and "pussy" are cute, but "cooter" or "cunt" are too raw.

> ## DIRTY DIALING
>
> If you want to try giving your honey some "lip," but you can't do it face-to-face, you might try something that's exciting, but keeps a little distance between you—a dirty phone call. For tips and pointers on this, check out the film *Obsession*, and play close attention to the part where the stalker, watching through a window nearby, calls the guy and tells him exactly where and when to touch himself. Mesmerized by her voice and the mysterious fact that she can see him but he can't see her, he does exactly as she says.

Remember that dirty talk doesn't have to represent what you'd say to each other out of bed, and Justin reminds you to keep it in context: "Sex is supposed to be exciting and fun and passionate. What happens in the bedroom stays in the bedroom—you can be as dirty and nasty as you want as long as you're both into it and know it's part of the fantasy." When the two of you know each other well, though, getting nasty from time to time can really help keep it fresh. As Bobby says, "If you can flip that switch, from soft and romantic to raunchy and randy, you can always keep her guessing. It will never get stale."

"You can talk about your fantasies during sex before actually enacting them," says Savanna, who admits she's not that verbal. Dirty talk is an opportunity for you to gauge your partner's interest in a particular fantasy. It can also be a safe way to test the waters before you buy the cheerleading uniform, take those tango lessons, or worse, invite the woman you met in Starbucks home for a threesome. Talk about that doctor-patient scenario or your sex-slave fantasy first, and see how your partner reacts. If something really works, you can ask later if the talk is as far as you want to take it, or if you're ready for the words to come to life.

As Chi Chi puts it, "You can be having everyday sex, but go off into another world by what you say." Imagine that you are stroking and stimulating your partner, but this time you're telling a story. Is he a captive on a planet of Amazons? Is she a princess being visited by her prince? Are you strangers who picked each other up at a bar? Not surprisingly, all three of our directors described this style of dirty talk. With words you can create fantasies and scenarios without actually doing anything different from what you usually do. Justin's style dates back to early erotic memories: "When I was young, I started masturbating to stories in magazines like *Penthouse Forum*. I am not as turned on by just pictures. I'm more of a storyteller, and I like fantasy scenarios. So talking dirty came very naturally to me. People should feel out their partners, discover what they fantasize about, then create a fantasy for them through words." Try weaving an erotic tale of your very own, or "borrow" one from an erotic novel or story and make it your own.

Vivid director Paul Thomas spices his sex life up this way: "When you're in a relationship, it's very difficult to be original and creative because you inevitably begin to repeat the same phrases and words. It's necessary to personalize it, to bring other people and events into it. In my relationship we don't see other people, but I'm still encouraging her to talk to me about men and women she sees and to 'lie' to me while I'm aroused, invent some outrageous situation that happened to her, like 'Did I tell you about the cabdriver I had today? Oh my God . . . ' And for the time being, I buy into it."

Stunning model Briana Banks is a twenty-three-year-old, long-legged, German-born beauty who walked out on a boring job as an insurance auditor to begin a career in adult entertainment and has never looked back. Born of a German mother and Italian father, Briana lived in Germany and England until she was seven, when her mother moved to Simi Valley, California. In high school she was a studious, shy kid who played volleyball and ran track (she still holds the school record at Royal High for the mile). She rarely dated and didn't even kiss a boy until she was seventeen. As a teenager, she was awarded custody of her younger sister. She graduated from high school living on child support, and held down jobs as a waitress and fashion model to pay for rent and groceries. "I was on the cover of *Teen* magazine, and thought I'd be a mainstream model. But it's such a competitive business, you go to auditions with dozens of other girls and hope they pick you. When I turned eighteen, I stopped getting that support check, and I was fired from my other job. Then I saw one of those ads, 'make a thousand dollars a day' to be in a film." So her career as an adult movie star began.

Briana got into the adult business when she was nineteen. "I always thought of myself as a skinny, dorky, giraffe-looking kid," Briana says. "Even though I had made the cover of *Teen* magazine as a model, I wasn't making any money. The day I quit my insurance job I got in a car accident and didn't even have enough cash to move my sister and me into an apartment from the room we had been renting, so I answered an ad in *L.A. Weekly* that said I could make up to a thousand dollars a day modeling. I had never even thought about porno, but I loved it. I guess I was sexually repressed.

"My first scene was in the movie *University Co-Eds,* and I called myself Mirage. I worked with Brandon Irons, and I remember when he pulled down his pants, I had never seen anything so big in all my life! He must have been ten inches! I was so nervous. I mean, I was the kind of girl who always had sex with the lights off. I was so self-conscious my first time on camera, I felt young and naive. Brandon was very gentle with me, but it was almost like losing my virginity all over again."

The inexperienced "Mirage" then had another deflowering of sorts: her first scene having sex with another woman. "My first girl-girl experience was with Lita Chase. I had always been curious about girls, but I had been too shy to try anything until I got into the business. Lita is a beautiful blonde with big breasts, and I was in awe of her. I had never touched such large boobs, and that was when I decided I wanted a pair of my own. Lita had me fly out to Florida to have her doctor perform the plastic surgery. When I had them done, it changed my image and I changed my name to Briana Banks. Having them done gave me so much more confidence. And the surgery also made my nipples more sensitive. Now my nipples will stand up even if someone just breathes on them."

Working in the adult industry transformed the self-described shy young woman: "Getting into the business, I have a new sexual freedom. I had never had sex with other people in the room, I wasn't used to being called pretty, and the whole experience has been very empowering. It's brought me out of my shell. Of course I still have insecurities, everyone does, but I am no longer timid. I really know my body better than I ever did before. I got my sex education on film, including my first orgasm, so my fans have watched me grow from a girl to a woman and I feel I have a very special relationship with them. Once into it, I decided I might as well do the best I could.

"Before long I got signed by Vivid, which is the pinnacle for anyone interested in erotic acting." Briana loves working with director Chi Chi LaRue: "Chi Chi is so awesome, and his movies are great. He is so fun to work with and his energy is reflected in the atmosphere on the set. He's so flamboyant and really loves his job. Plus, he genuinely cares about his actresses." Briana likes working for Vivid because she really feels like part of a family, and "I get to have sex with men who really know what they are doing. And I get to play fun parts. I played a sex therapist who listened to people's erotic fantasies and dilemmas. Vivid has such strong story lines—I get to play a punk-rock star next!"

Briana graced the cover of the June 2001 issue of *Penthouse,* and was nominated as the 2002 Penthouse Pet of the Year after readers flipped over a twelve-page pictorial and centerfold shot by famed photographer Earl Miller. Also in 2002 she made *Briana Loves Jenna* with top porn star Jenna Jameson and the movie went on to become the best selling and renting adult video of the year. "When I shot *Briana Loves Jenna,* I had so much fun. I like girls, Jenna is gorgeous, we were all over each other, and we had the best time. When I shot *She Devil,* I was hanging off the edge of the fire escape on the top floor of a thirteen-story building while having sex. It was terrifying, but that also added to the intensity of the sex."

When her adult acting career is over, she wants to go behind the scenes to start her own line of adult movies, work on her website, and return to college full-time. Meanwhile, she works out every day, paying special attention to a boxing and weight-lifting routine she has developed. She also indulges in her favorite sports—motocross racing, surfing, and

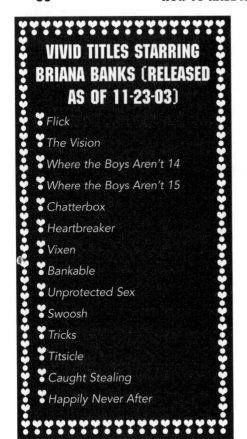

VIVID TITLES STARRING BRIANA BANKS (RELEASED AS OF 11-23-03)

- Flick
- The Vision
- Where the Boys Aren't 14
- Where the Boys Aren't 15
- Chatterbox
- Heartbreaker
- Vixen
- Bankable
- Unprotected Sex
- Swoosh
- Tricks
- Titsicle
- Caught Stealing
- Happily Never After

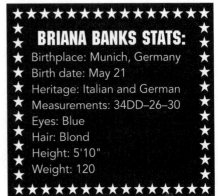

BRIANA BANKS STATS:
- Birthplace: Munich, Germany
- Birth date: May 21
- Heritage: Italian and German
- Measurements: 34DD–26–30
- Eyes: Blue
- Hair: Blond
- Height: 5'10"
- Weight: 120

snowboarding. Sims Snowboards will introduce two Briana Banks boards with images of her clothed and nude in its Fader line this year.

Born in May, this Taurus's favorite movies include *Casino*, *Scarface*, and *Kingpin*. She loves the Dave Matthews Band and Linkin Park, and thinks it's great to have sex while listening to Prodigy or Nine Inch Nails. And where does she think the sexiest hot spot in the house is? "The bathroom is fun. But I have broken more towel racks than you can imagine! I end up using one for leverage, and it snaps right off the wall!"

4
adjust those headlights

Fantasy File:

    Bored and disappointed with her yuppie married sex life, the girl drives to a place she's never been to before—someplace very out of character, almost dangerous. Even before she opens the door to the run-down storefront on the rough side of town, she hears the steady beat of rock music blaring from the jukebox inside. Taking a deep breath, she opens the door and walks straight to the bar, past tables filled with biker guys and their women friends drinking beer. The bartender asks, "What'll you have?" "I think I'm in the mood for something different," the girl exclaims. Hearing this, one of the bikers and his girlfriend at the bar respond, "So are we."

    The biker motions to the bartender to bring over a bottle, and pours shots for three of them. The girl notices how stunning the biker's girlfriend looks, with her long blond hair streaming straight down, black leather shorts over a high round ass, and a tight T-shirt showing off her large, perfectly shaped breasts. It's only a matter of moments before the alcohol begins to loosen her inhibitions. She locks eyes with the blonde, whose fingers begin massaging her leg. The two girls begin to dance slowly together in a corner of the bar where two show bikes are parked. One of the bikers lifts his beer, looks in their direction, and says something inaudible to his companions. The blond biker girl rubs her hands up and down the other girl's arms and quietly begins to lick them. She circles behind the girl, cups her breasts, caresses them, kneading their forms in her hands. The girl sighs deeply, her bosom swelling inside the satin bra with each breath she takes. The women begin to lick and kiss each other, first on the cheek, and then fully on the mouth. Slowly, almost in time with the music, the blonde pushes the girl ever so slightly back onto the chopper, lays her head on the handlebars, and climbs up on top of her. The girl's long brown hair falls into a curtain, as the slow, sensual licking continues and both shirts drop silently to the floor. The smell of the warm worn leather arouses her as it brushes against her tingling skin. She looks down between her own pointed breasts, where a tangle of blond hair sways back and forth as the biker girl's talented tongue navigates below the top of her bra. She wants to reach out and touch the voluminous breasts pressed close to her, but she is consumed with desire now, desperately wanting and needing to be touched. The blonde's breasts fall on her like soft mountains enveloped in clouds. She feels like she's dreaming. From where she lay under them, she longs to take them in her mouth and suck them. Without words, the biker girl removes both their bras, freeing their breasts from their confinement, the girl's skirt, and, finally, her own leather shorts. The girl squeezes the blonde's ass with both hands. The other responds by squeezing the tips of the girl's breasts with her thumb and forefinger. Even as her nipples become pointed and hard, the blonde's caresses are relentless. "Hey, sexy girl," the blonde says, looking up into the wells of her black eyes and, for a second, unclasping her nipples long enough to stroke her dark brown hair. They smile and close their eyes again in pleasure. Returning to the girl's sensual body, the biker girl slowly massages the girl's clit with a determined, circular movement. "Oh," the girl moans. "Oh, yes. Please." With her other hand the biker girl reverently continues to stroke the girl's breasts and pinch her nipples. Suddenly the girl cannot wait any longer. In a gesture of wild abandon, she leans back farther and extends her legs up in the air into an open V while the blonde instinctively steadies one leg between her heaving breasts. Hungrily, the blonde makes her way down to the soft lips of the girl's pussy. She spreads the wet lips apart with one hand while the other hand remains on the girl's breast, turning and twisting the nipple between her fingers. The biker guy, filled with desire from the sight of their tender lovemaking, slams back another shot, wipes his arm on the bandanna wrapped around his head, and saunters over to the two girls. "So how was she, baby?" he asks his girlfriend as he pats her firm ass. The blonde smiles at him. The biker inserts his finger into the girl's open pussy to feel how ready she is for more, and begins to loosen his belt buckle.

★★ *from* Rolling Thunder,
directed by Derrick Lane

Breasts: Your Own and Your Partner's

What is it about women's breasts that makes all men go nuts? Perhaps it harkens back to infancy when baby boys were suckled at their mothers' bosoms? Could it be that when men come face-to-face with breasts some mysterious instinctive force takes over and they just want to grab them? Or could it be that guys are particularly mesmerized by women's breasts because, size-wise, women's blow men's out of the water? Whatever the reason, guys are drawn to breasts like moths to a flame. But they're no longer infants, and it should be obvious that a six-foot-tall, 175-pound man (who may or may not have rough stubble on his face) should exercise care when dealing with these glorious globes. "Men get overexcited when they see big boobs and they just want to mangle them," says Mercedez. "To that I say, hey, would you want me to mangle your balls because I like how they look?" In all seriousness, Mercedez makes a valid point. There are so many nicknames for breasts that seem to imply that they're playthings to flip around like pancakes: knockers, hooters, juggies, knobs, bazoombas, balloons, and kahoonas, to name a few. But in Vivid movies, a woman's breasts are never treated casually or carelessly.

Before getting into specific advice about breast handling, we want to emphasize that breast play can be very exciting for men and women alike. Some people are really into it, and others can take it or leave it. Without getting into a whole anatomy course, let's just say that in order to know what might be pleasurable to the opposite sex, it's important to have a good sense of the way they're built. For both genders, the nipples are the most sensitive parts. (More on this later.) To arouse a man's breasts, women can begin with a tantalizing massage of the chest area around the nipples and move inward. Guys who work out are often more aware of their pectoral muscles, so everything feels more sensitive for them. Women's breasts, on the other hand, are full of milk glands and other sensitive tissue, so they require a lighter touch. Men should also begin with the outermost areas and move in toward the nipples, but the touch must be much softer and delicate; and absolutely no slapping them around!

Breasts are a big deal in the adult industry. According to Chi Chi, "Breasts are very important to the look of a movie" But the experiences of our stars reveal that many men, although they love to look at them, aren't so sure how to handle them in real life. Working a woman's breasts and nipples is one skill every lover should master. Some women, if their breasts are teased or touched in just the right way, can approach orgasm from that alone. For other women, even if they are not quite that sensitive, breast play is essential to getting the juices flowing. Here, the owners of some of the most prized and admired bosoms in the world reveal how they like them touched, handled, and licked.

The Right Way to Play

"I like my breasts touched softly; grabbing them really hard is not sexy and doesn't feel good," says Mercedez. Just about all women would agree. "I don't like when they grab too hard," says Dasha. "Be gentle, be soft, go slow." The pleasurable nerve endings are all right on the surface of the skin, so a very light touch is all you need to get started. Tawny's nipples are extremely responsive: "My nipples are su-persensitive, so I don't like them pulled or pinched—just very softly played with." One caress that works for some women is for the man to spread out his fingers until they touch her skin lightly. Then draw them together as you pull your hand back so that the touch remains light across her skin and, perhaps, just grazing her nipple at the last moment. As you open and close your hand to repeat the motion, it will look like a butterfly opening and closing its wings. Only this particular butterfly will send her into flights of ecstasy. This motion works particularly well on small- to medium-size breasts because a man's hand can usually take in the entire area. For big-busted women, try cupping them from underneath, then move up, drawing your thumb and fingers together gently as you approach the nipples.

> **" It's great when you find a girl who has very sensitive breasts. Judging their sensitivity should determine how you treat them. If they're very sensitive, use very light touches. "**
>
> —Justin

Another movement is to trace a spiral inward with your finger-tip, starting at the edge of her breast and ending at her nipple. If your caresses are having an effect, her nipple will harden. If you are in the right position for it, use both hands on both breasts simultaneously. This is a great tease, as the nipple is more sensitive than the rest of the breast and the sensation heightens the closer your finger comes to it.

This is foreplay, so vary your positions. Rather than approach-ing them head-on, sometimes it's sexier to come up from behind, kiss her neck, and fondle her breasts. And while you're playing with her breasts, it's important to look up at her from time to time, if not to maintain eye contact constantly. You want to make sure she doesn't feel that you're more into her breasts than you are into her! You also need to read her reactions as you touch her. When you intensify your touch, centering on the nipple, you may see her expression change.

Nipples

❝ ❝ I had my nipples pierced and it made them sensitive. I love to watch the lips of my partner on my nipples. ❞ ❞

—*Savanna*

One way to start out on the nipple is to let your fingers do the walking. Using your index and middle fingers of each hand, alternate one after the other with a "walking" or twiddling motion of your fingertips, gently squeezing across the tip of the nipple. If she responds to this, apply more pressure, or move your fingers faster. Another method is to twist the nipples with a gentle tweak using your thumb and index finger. Apply light pressure at first. If your partner seems to like it with more intensity, or if he or she needs a firmer touch, squeeze and twist your fingers together harder. Some people like their nipples handled a little rougher. Just remember to go slowly so you don't rub them raw. And always use small twisting or rubbing movements. It goes without saying that if your partner's nipples are pierced like Savanna's, they are much more sensitive, and it's a good guess that he or she is definitely into nipple play. But be careful. There are a few people with piercings who like to have their nipple rings tugged on gently. But for the most part, we suggest you concentrate on the nipple itself and avoid the hardware unless told otherwise.

Tweaking

An extension of twisting is tweaking, and you can see excellent examples of this in *Where the Boys Aren't 14, Where the Boys Aren't 15,* and *Blondage.* Tweaking is like a soft little pinch done with your thumb and forefinger. You can use this motion to help encourage your partner's nipples to go from soft to hard, or you can use it when the nipples are already hard and your partner wants you to increase the pressure. When the nipples are soft, it's okay to gently pinch the slightly larger area that includes the areola—the darker circle around the tip. But when the nipples are rock hard, it will be more exciting if you just tweak the tip. Women should try this on guys, too. Most men have some sensation in their nipples, and some are extremely sensitive. "I know some men who love to have their nipples played with or pinched—sometimes very hard," says Chi Chi. But be aware that a fair number of men are just the opposite, and tweaking their nipples won't do a thing for them.

Dasha says she likes her nipples handled a little harder than most women: "A lot of guys don't really know how to play with the nipples. I like kissing, using just a little bit of teeth sliding through but not too hard. With me they are not that sensitive and I like a little pinching and twisting because I can really feel it. A little bit of the tongue while kissing the nipples—I can't really feel it, so it has to be a little harder for me than [for] other women." If your partner likes it on the rougher side, like Dasha, start with the tweaking motion, and once you get a good grip, pull on the nipple. Pull it toward you, twist it, and roll the nipple between your fingers all at the same time.

Handle It Yourself

Often, when women are masturbating, they will massage their own breasts and tweak or tug their own nipples. If her partner doesn't have enough hands, or if those hands are busy elsewhere, a woman might fondle herself while her partner is going down on her, or even during intercourse. For guys, this is an excellent time to watch how a woman handles her own breasts because you can see what she likes best, and when. Good self-handling scenes can be seen in *Savanna Superstar* as well as in *Where the Boys Aren't 14* and *Where the Boys Aren't 15.*

Wet Fingers

Another approach is to lick your finger and then circle the tip of her nipples with the wet fingertip, as Justin recommends. There's a good example of this in the first sex sequence of *Rolling Thunder*. "Use a little saliva on your finger, on the tip," says Justin, "and then when you go down for the kiss, it's very important to keep eye contact with her." Blow gently on the wet nipples. If they are not already hard, they will be when you're through. If they are already hard, they may get even harder!

Licking

The natural extension of wetting her nipple with your finger is to use your tongue directly on it. You can lap at her nipples softly like a cat, draw circles around them with the tip of your tongue, or flick them up and down with rapid fluttering motions. She will feel a wonderful contrast between the warmth of your tongue with the coolness of your saliva. Take a break from time to time to gently blow on them as well. Justin has some more hints for using your mouth. "Don't stay on one nipple too long, and always touch the other nipple while you're sucking one. You don't want her to get one-sided, or leave one side feeling neglected."

Sucking

Of course you can draw the nipple into your mouth by sucking on it. There's a great nipple scene in *Bangkok Nights* with a sailor and his paid companion, who gives him a sponge bath. If by this time you've discovered that she likes it harder and rougher, you can suck pretty hard. Sucking on the nipple draws blood to the surface, which can increase sensitivity, so after you suck on them, try blowing on them, or rubbing them lightly with your fingertips. For Kira, finding out what kind of stimulation she liked was a matter of experimentation: "I used to say, 'They're for display only; don't touch 'em.' But now I say suck on them, lick them, play with them! My current partner, he experimented a lot, and now he's gotten it right. He barely licks them, then sucks them lightly. Then, once he's got me so turned on, he can play with them harder."

Biting and Teething

Justin says, "There's nothing wrong with biting them as long as she's into it. You have to test it first. Give a little nibble; if you see them give a moan and a gasp then you know you're going in the right direction." Use caution when using your teeth. It can be quite exciting to use them to graze the nipple rather than bite down right away. If you do bite down, try it first with your lips over your teeth, and just squeeze the flesh that way. You can bite down harder, using your bare teeth, if she really likes it, but in general you cannot bite down with serious force.

Some women also love the sensation of having the main part of their breasts, not just the nipples, nibbled. "I like having my breasts and nipples sucked on, and if I'm in the mood, bitten. When he swirls his tongue around my nipple, then pulls away, teasing me, that's the best!" says Briana. Also experiment with *lightly* holding the nipple between your top and bottom teeth while you lick with the tip of your tongue to add to the excitement.

Vibrator on Nipples

You'll notice in certain films, *Obsession* for example, a vibrator may be applied to the breasts. Doing this is not only a matter of personal preference, it also depends on the type of vibrator you're using. Most of the time in the films, the vibrators that are used on the nipples are not the really powerful ones, but the gentler battery-powered models used on low speed. The only thing to remember is never to push the vibrator into the breast, which could become painful. Just a little buzz on the nipple will be scintillating.

Titty Fucking

This very visual maneuver is seen in several movies, among them *Domination Nation*. "I love when a guy slides his penis between a pair," says Chi Chi. A common image in adult movies, this move may seem more for the enjoyment of the man, but some women enjoy the sensation as well. No matter what size your breasts are, a woman can squeeze them together to make a nice soft tunnel for his penis to go through. Lots of men enjoy the visual this creates as well as the sensation. Use lube for a smooth, slick motion that's comfortable for both of you. And when a guy comes from sliding his penis between a woman's breasts, it's called "squeezing for dollars." If a man is particularly well endowed, he should be careful not to thrust too hard or close to the woman's neck, which can be very annoying.

Wet 'n Wild

Saliva isn't the only substance that can be used on nipples. An ice cube can be great on a hot summer night, but only if the cube is slightly melted so that it slides back and forth easily. In *Blondage* and *Where the Boys Aren't 15,* champagne is festively squirted all over the breasts and then licked off. In *Obsession,* as well as in some other films, couples who are outdoors use cold water from a garden hose. Cold water against warm breasts is a surefire way to get the nipples hard and keep them that way. Some people enjoy the idea of licking whipped cream, honey, or chocolate syrup off the breasts, and there's a part in *Intimate Journey* where a woman excites herself by doing this. For the messier of these liquid maneuvers, it goes without saying that they should be done either outdoors, or in places like bathrooms and kitchens, where postcoital cleanup is easier, and where you won't have to sleep on wet, sticky sheets afterward.

Other ORBits

There are just a few more things you might have seen on-screen that we'd like to mention here. Earlier in this chapter, we specifically said "no slapping," but in certain films, such as *Looking In,* you might see something we'll call "paddling." The difference between the two is, basically, that when a woman has larger breasts, her partner can gently move them from side to side rhythmically, as long as it doesn't hurt her (and as long as it doesn't turn into a paddleball game). The same thing goes for something we'll call "kneading." Just remember this isn't the local baking contest, so keep your breast kneading light. Although the Vivid Girls generally recommend a softer touch, if your partner enjoys a vigorous breast massage, go right ahead.

Finally, something you see in many adult movies is what's called "a pearl necklace." This is when a woman squeezes her breasts together and the man ejaculates on them. While most women don't often suggest this to their partners, they would be thrilled to comply if they knew how much visual pleasure this move offers men. As we've said many times, communication is key. So if this is something you've seen on the screen and want to try, why not bring it up during pillow talk?

Up Close & Personal
★ Kira Kener ★

"If you're doing it in a limo, just make sure you know when you're coming to your stop so you don't get surprised by the driver." Only someone who is as down-to-earth about wild sex would give the advice Kira Kener does. But she wasn't always so uninhibited or adventurous. The petite five-foot four-inch Eurasian beauty was born to a Vietnamese mother and Norwegian father and was raised in San Jose, California. Kira describes her unlikely journey to adult movie superstardom while she was living in North Carolina. "I was absolutely the most naive person on the planet. I had never seen a porn movie before. I thought the Dollhouse (a local strip club) was an upscale antique store until I applied for a job as a cocktail waitress." When she "got the nerve" to move from waitress to dancer, a new world opened up for her.

Kira entered the adult entertainment industry as a topless dancer, performing at clubs around the country. Before long, she had become a headliner at famous spots such as the Crazy Horse Gentlemen's Club in San Francisco and the Spearmint Rhino in Southern California. Her accomplishments on the dance stage have earned her numerous top honors, including Miss Nude Asia 1997 and 1998, 1998's Best Stage Performer, and Exotic Dancer Cover Girl of the Year. As a dancer, she got the opportunity to meet feature dancers from all over the country, and many of them were Vivid contract performers. "They were beautiful, they had amazing stage presence, and they had all these fans." In fact, it was while Kira was performing at a club on the East Coast that another dancer who had worked in adult movies suggested that she contact Vivid Entertainment. She was signed to an exclusive, multiple-movie contract and Vivid named her as one of the celebrated Vivid Girls. Her first movie with Vivid was the 1999 release *Nurses*.

When she joined Vivid in 1999, Kira's first job was filming two movies back-to-back: *Nurses* and *The Window*. "The first day on the set, I saw Julian lying on a bed naked, and I thought, 'Oh my God, are all the male performers that well endowed?' He looked huge to me. I was so shy, and I didn't know anything at all. When Julian went down on me during our scene, a lightbulb went off; I finally realized what all the fuss about oral sex was! I squealed, it felt so good."

That was one of the many new experiences Kira would soon have, and she admits that she had her very first orgasm on the set of a movie. "I learned pretty much everything I know now about sex on the set of adult movies. Having somebody pull my hands over my head so I felt like I had no control, talking dirty, even anal sex—these are all things that I tried first in movies, then incorporated into my sex life at home."

Watching magicians perform their wonders may be one of her hobbies offscreen, but Kira certainly creates her own magic on screen. Kira likes working with different directors because she enjoys "seeing their unique vision, the world through their eyes." One of her favorites is Paul Thomas: "I love working with Paul because he really understands me. He was the first to shoot me, and he gave me so much advice. He's an experienced actor and director, and he really taught me how to communicate with a director. Now that I have those skills, I like working with all of the directors. They have all taught me so much."

Kira believes that adult movies can have a teaching function, as they inspire viewers to try new things. "Look at how many people copy mainstream movies," she says, "like *9½ Weeks*—the ice cubes, the striptease, the public sex. People see things in adult movies and they want to try them."

When Kira began working for Vivid, her outlook on sex expanded greatly. Now she is the one expanding her partner's view. "My new man, he's been pretty conservative all this time, because he was in a long relationship where sex was just boring. You always have to be creative or it's going to get dull." And where is this beauty's favorite sexy hot spot? "I love to have sex in the rain or in the shower. Everything is wet, and it feels so fantastic." Commenting on her favorite background music for sex, Kira says, "There definitely needs to be something in Keith Sweat, ballads, or eighties rock. I'm also a huge Kiss fan."

Kira says her most memorable movie scene was with Nick Manning in a film called *Frosted*. "We have a chemistry that I haven't come across with any other performer I have worked with . . . We flirt with each other, and we both push each other's buttons in a good way. After the scene, he left my legs quivering, and I was ready to pass out. He just really outdid himself."

Kira keeps things from getting dull with her wardrobe, too. "I have my moods, but whatever I wear it's going to be sexy. I always wear heels. I can't go without heels. It would depend on where we were going on a date, but it's definitely going to be something tight, whether leather and a short top, or a dress. At home, I run around in the house in lingerie. I'll run around in a corset regularly; I love it! And every man loves heels. It makes your legs look sexy, they make you feel sexy. I keep my heels on to have sex."

Her man appreciates the efforts she goes to, and gives back to her tenfold. "I've been so open with him, it's so amazing. I'm loving him touching my nipples, which I never liked before, and it's just that everything gets better and better. When you think you've had it all, you suddenly discover new things. Being with the right person makes all the difference in the world, because even though we've done it so many times before, he can still touch spots inside of me that I never knew existed."

In March 2002 Kira appeared in the *Playboy* magazine "Sizzling Porn Star Pictorial" gracing the cover along with Vivid Girl Dasha. Most recently, she was chosen as the December 2002 *Penthouse* Pet of the Month and was the subject of a lavish pictorial in the magazine. True to her astrological sign, Leo, Kira is open, honest, and fun loving, and her favorite movie of all time is *Pretty Woman.* Asked what kind of man she likes, she jokes that she loves older men with gray hair and a beer belly. (Not!)

With her exotic good looks and her erotic on-screen performances, Kira is destined for stardom in the adult world!

VIVID FEATURES STARRING KIRA KENER (RELEASED AS OF 11-25-03)

- Nurses
- The Window
- Housesitter
- The Bet
- Rue Blue
- Façade
- Return to Sender
- Obsession
- Eye Spy
- Prisoner
- Innervision
- Breathe
- Thrills
- Thrills 2
- Where the Boys Aren't 14
- Where the Boys Aren't 15
- Open All Night
- The Scent
- ECU: Kira Kener
- 20 Candles
- Moxie
- Sexual Misbehavior
- White Room
- The Arrangement
- Reflections in a Window
- C-Men #1
- Swirl
- Unfinished
- Any Dorm in a Storm
- Virtual Love
- Hollywood Hostel
- Ms. Fortune
- Rack 'Em

KIRA KENER STATS:

- Birthplace: San Jose, CA
- Birth date: August 11
- Ethnic Heritage: Norwegian-Vietnamese
- Measurements: 34DD–24–28
- Eyes: Light Brown
- Hair: Brown
- Height: 5'4"
- Weight: 113
- Hobbies: Fashion design, relaxation, special f/x, watching magicians

Kira Kener Fan Club:
2054 Kildaire Farm Road #354
Cary, NC 27511

5
going down (on her)

Fantasy File:

The techno music pumps at a loud, feverish pitch at Jenna's Underground, the all-superstar girlie bar. On one side, a long, lean, blond bombshell and a dark-haired shoeshine vixen start the evening off right.

"Suck, my slave," orders the blonde.

The hired help gets right down to work, spreading the blonde's porcelain thighs apart and diving right onto her pussy. She licks up and down steadily, covering the area with wet, glistening saliva before turning her full attention to the quivering clit. Overcome with passion, the blonde reaches down and rapidly pounds two fingers in and out of her own pussy while the shoeshine girl alternates between tapping the other's clit and rubbing it between her fingers.

They switch places so that the blonde has a full view of the girl's ass and pussy from behind. She slaps the girl's ass a few times to "prime the pump," and teases her hungry pussy and asshole with her mouth. As the blonde rubs the girl's pussy up and down and sideways, a third glamorous beauty saunters over. "How do you like my boys?" asks Jenna, the proprietor, as she strolls in front of elevated boxes on which several guys are dancing. The go-go guys are the ne plus ultra of hard bodies, tight asses, and oversize packages. "I like to keep dick in my bar. It gets my other side going, plus it turns the girls on to turn the boys on." Jenna walks in front of another beautiful blonde leaning back on a full-size birdcage with a go-go guy inside. "We play a little game," Jenna continues. "We try to get them up. The girls like to get them excited, but if one of them steps off the boxes, he's fired."

As the boys dance in the background, Jenna, looking hot in her sexy tight tank top, rubs her firm breasts back and forth on the girl's abundant ass. Then she coaxes her to lie down. With masterful technique, Jenna works up a mouthful of saliva and spits it on the girl's open pussy. She uses her fingertips to rub the girl's hardening clit, and darts her pointed tongue in and out of her salubrious slit. "Oh, oh," moans the girl as she throws her head back with pleasure. She grabs the wild mane of hair of her tender tormentor and grinds Jenna's face into her humping mound. Without a word, Jenna flips this morsel over onto her stomach, spreads her cheeks, and works up another mouthful of saliva. She lets it go, right on the girl's anus, and begins licking it furiously while she pokes one finger in and out of her pussy. As the girl screams out in ecstasy, something else attracts Jenna's attention.

Three voluptuous young starlets are looking for some fun. Removing their panties, they lean back on a platform in front of the boxes, and raise their shapely legs in the air to taunt the dancers. One by one, the dancers grasp the girls by their ankles and spread their legs apart, exposing three pulsating pussies and anticipating assholes for all to see. It is now up to Jenna to fulfill her role as the perfect nightclub hostess, and to ensure the pleasure of all three of her newest patrons.

★★ *From* Where the Boys Aren't 14, *directed by Chi Chi LaRue*

Oral Explorer

There's nothing like having your face between a gal's legs to really get in touch with her private parts. Women appreciate enthusiastic, skill-ful oral sex as much as men love a good blow job. Oral sex can be a tease, part of foreplay, or the main activity of the night. Many women say that cunnilingus is their favorite thing and the easiest way for them to have an orgasm. "I prefer a tongue to fingers," Sunrise says. "Fingers just don't feel right to me, but I like the tongue. It's warm, and it can be hard or soft." The Vivid team knows plenty about what it takes to lick a leading lady right, and they share their secrets throughout this chapter.

❝❝ I can have an orgasm without any fingers or penetration if my clit is being worked properly. Be really aware of it, become one with it. You can really feel it and feel what's going on there. ❞❞

—*Savanna*

When it comes to lapping between her legs, different women like different techniques. Some prefer a light flicking of the tongue, others crave broad strokes or a circular motion, while still others like firm movements or even sucking. And just like a man, women usually prefer a lighter movement in the beginning, other movements to sustain and increase their arousal, and yet a third, more determined movement as they come into the home stretch. The better you get to know your partner's parts as well as her individual preferences, the better you'll be able to please her.

One thing almost all women have in common is the process their bodies go through when they get turned on. When a woman is aroused, blood rushes to her genitals and the tissue becomes engorged. Her outer and inner lips swell, her vagina begins to lubricate, and her clitoris (which is made of erectile tissue like the penis) gets erect and becomes more pronounced, thus easier to find. All parts of her genitals become more sensitive, especially the clitoris, which retreats behind the flap of tissue around it called the clitoral hood. With thousands of nerve endings, the clitoris is the most sensitive part of a woman's body. Needless to say, wet and slippery oral stimulation feels great on such a receptive body part.

Oral stimulation can start before she even undresses. Place one hand on each of her thighs and position your head between her legs. Open your mouth wide and bring it close to her underwear—exhale slowly. The warm air will feel delicious through the cloth of her panties. To tease her more, with her underwear still on, use your lips to rub and nibble all over her pubic area. All the teasing will heighten her arousal and her need to be touched directly. Bobby prides himself on his ability to tease and torment a woman: "I like to kiss her and touch her all over, get her all hot and bothered, and then inch my way down near her pussy and tease her a bit. I'll lick her legs, her thighs, and just when she's trying to bury my face in her pussy, I'll go up and kiss her mouth some more." Briana loves to be tantalized, too: "Tease her right over her underwear, then slide it to one side, lick her outer lips, her inner lips, tease her a lot."

There's some great scenes of preliminary tongue teasing over underwear in *Where the Boys Aren't 14*. Dasha, looking totally hot in punky fishnets, a black belt and panties, and sequined pasties on her nipples, is sitting in a high chair getting her patent-leather boots polished by a comely shoeshine girl wearing little more than tighty-whitey BVDs. First she puts the pointy toe of her boot between the girl's legs and rubs in and out a bit to get the juices flowing. At one point, Dasha gets down from the chair, gets behind the girl, and, over her panties, slowly runs her tongue up the girl's ass crack from bottom to top. When the girl is sufficiently aroused, Dasha rips the crotch of her white panties apart and begins to lick under the panties.

Close Shave

We've already talked about shaving or waxing one's privates, but it goes without saying that a woman's genital area is supersensitive. No matter how talented a guy is with his tongue, it's going to be uncomfortable for the woman if his rough stubble is rubbing on her vaginal lips or inner thighs. So follow Tawny's advice and "shave before bedtime." Justin reiterates this. "If you don't have a goatee, make sure you're shaven." And we'll also add, even if you have a goatee, you might want to think about using some simple hair conditioner to soften it. And girls, it goes without saying that you should be washed and freshly fragrant.

Good Timing

There are those who eat to live, and those who live to eat. And to continue the analogy, some people rush through meals to get on with something else, and others savor each course to make a good meal last. We highly recommend viewing some scenes from two films, *Suite 18* and *Good Things,* to get a good look at gourmet action. A good meal should never be rushed.

In *Suite 18,* a man in a business suit gets it on with a girl in a hotel room. The guy works his kisses down, beginning with the breasts and landing on the girl's pussy. She leans back with her legs apart and plays with his hair while he's down there. The businessman concentrates on using his mouth for a substantial period of time, adding a finger inside sporadically. He gets his nose right in there, starting with smooth lapping, then uses the tip of his tongue to move back and forth slowly between her ass and her clit. What's great about this scene is that it demonstrates some extended tongue action within a realistic time frame. Men should remember that it takes women longer than men to get aroused, and usually a longer time for them to reach an orgasm. If a guy wants the woman to come from oral action before moving on to other things, he must commit the time to do the job right.

Good Things is filled with hot oral scenes. In one, the heroine watches a porn flick on TV in which a woman is on top of a guy in a reverse-69-type position. She lowers her rear onto his face while giving him a BJ. But what's worthy of mention is the way the guy gets his mouth right up there on her clit. Another scene is supposedly also on TV. The heroine watches Sunrise lie back with her legs spread while a guy goes down on her. He stretches back the skin of her pubic mound, not only to give himself a clearer shot of her clit, but also because this helps direct the sensation toward her clit, and increases her awareness of the whole vaginal area. He deliberately licks and laps up and down slowly, first on her vagina, then on her clit. As she gets more excited, he increases the pace. Again, this scene is great because the guy takes his time to pleasure the woman before going on to another course. A third scene between the heroine's sister and a neighbor illustrates another interesting pose. He's on his back and she's on top with her right knee bent down on the bed, and her left knee bent up so that her foot is near the left side of his head. The neighbor guy takes his time drawing lazy circles on the girl's vaginal lips, and then proceeds to do the same motion on her clit.

Basic Techniques

❝ ❝ **It's really important for a man to communicate with her, to ask what technique she likes. There are so many ways to do it, and every girl is different. ❞ ❞**

—Jenna

Once her underwear is off, your journey to her sexual center can intensify. When you first start to go down on a woman, experimentation is key. Be aware that there are several things you can vary: body positions, tongue movements and rhythms, hand actions, which part(s) you lick, and for how long. First off, women don't usually like guys to dive in; they liked to be teased a little. Like the businessman in *Suite 18,* work your way toward her genital area. You can start downward with kisses and licks to her lips, neck, breasts, tummy, and inner thighs. Or, you can start upward beginning with her toes, the sensitive soles of the feet, inside her knees, and up to her inner thighs.

Lick her inner and outer lips, her opening, her clitoris, the area around her anus, and try a bunch of different techniques for each. See how her body responds to your stimulation. Does she like it light and gentle or firm? Your lips on her lips (her other lips, we should say) are a great tease. Begin slowly and lightly with a few flicks of your tongue; she will be expecting you to go straight for the clit, but you can make her wait by circling around it, nibbling and tugging softly on the loose folds of her vagina with your mouth. When you work your way to her clit, try creating different sensations with your tongue on that very sensitive spot; flick it back and forth, make a circular motion, or lick it from top to bottom.

As you continue to experiment, try using the wide middle of your tongue (instead of just the tip), where it is wettest and softest. You can rub this any which way over the clit, licking upward, in a circle, or by moving your whole head from side to side. The center of the tongue feels quite different from the muscular, pointy tip of the tongue. Mercedez prefers this method: "Some guys do a thing where they get their tongue really hard in the front and it doesn't work for me. It's better when you stick your tongue out if it is relaxed. I like that part of his tongue moving in a circle. I can definitely come from soft licking if it's done right." Flutter your tongue, touching the clit as lightly as possible at first, and then increase the pressure. You can vary the pressure and intensity both by how hard you move your tongue against her, and also by positioning your head up and down her most sensitive areas. But whatever you do, listen to her moans and don't change positions abruptly. Often, a woman needs sustained stimulation to one specific area of her clit to raise her level of excitement.

Savanna agrees with Mercedez, and reminds men that when you are getting started, the clit isn't completely aroused or erect yet, and it is often at its most sensitive and vulnerable then, so be careful. "I don't like it too hard," says Savanna. "Some guys think they really have to work you hard! At first, do it really lightly with soft strokes. When the clit gets hard and swollen, then you can work it harder. I think guys should err on the side of being gentle, and she can always grab his head and grind it in harder. It depends on the clit. You have to be really aware of the stages of arousal it goes through—it changes so much during a sexual encounter." Savanna is absolutely right: give your woman a chance to get turned on before you move on to firmer or more focused stimulation with your tongue.

One more word of caution: whatever you do, don't confuse little nibbles with your lips with biting with your teeth. Says Mercedez, "Once I was dancing in a club and ended up bringing this guy to my room afterward. It ended up being the worst thing. He was down there way too long, biting it. He really didn't know what he was doing. Men who don't know how to give oral should be banned!"

Body Positions

Adjusting who's where and at what angle can change the whole experience for both of you. The basic position has the woman on her back with the guy's head between her legs. In this position, some women like to have their legs out straight, some like them bent up or out, some like them wrapped around their partner's back, and some like them straight up in the air—or a combination of all these at different times. To make yourself more comfortable for the long haul, and to make access to her genital area easier, you don't want your chin digging into the mattress or to have a stiff neck in the morning. You can raise her bottom up on pillows, which will work nicely. Or, try positioning her so that her rear is at the edge of the bed, chair, or dining-room table, with her feet bent up or flat down on the floor; you sit on the floor between her legs. This is the position the businessman used in *Suite 18,* and it's basically the same position used by the shoeshine girl with Dasha in a high chair in *Where the Boys Aren't 14.*

The second group of positions are all variations that have the woman on top, either with her head facing the guy's feet, as in the porn video in *Good Things,* or with her head facing the same way as his. The advantage of head to toe is that the woman can use her mouth on the guy at the same time. This is also a variation on the usual 69 position, where people go down on each other lying side by side. You can see another really good scene of 69 in *Chasey Loves Rocco.* Another woman-on-top position in *Good Times* has her head higher than his, with one leg bent up so she can lower herself onto his mouth. A variation on this is where the woman stands with her legs spread apart and her partner sits between them licking upward. You'll see a lot of this stance in adult movies because it affords the camera person a good shot. And there's one other variation that requires a lightweight girl and a very strong guy. This is where the man lifts the woman in the air by her waist, and twirls her upside down. If she starts off facing him, she can go down on him while locking her thighs on his shoulders. If she starts facing away from him, he'll have better access to her ass and pussy, but he has to be really strong to hold her that way for any length of time. Plus, you can both lose your balance easily, so you might want to test this position with the guy leaning against a wall. If you're interested in trying this really awesome 69 position, check out the Emperor and the concubine in the last scenes of *Lotus*. Or try it out while lying flat first before you tackle the more demanding aerial gymnastics.

Where to Lick

We've already talked about the importance of extended licking time, but we haven't talked specifically about where to lick. Some women love tongue inside the opening of their vagina, or inside the labial folds, while, for others, this does very little. Some women like to be licked around and just inside their ass opening, which is called rimming. This is especially good as a prelude to anal sex, or finger insertion, but it also can be exciting in and of itself. However, other women may be squeamish about this, or not like it at all; so do experiment. Again, the Vivid crew unanimously agrees that all women like to have their clits licked, so that should definitely be the focus of your attention.

Tongue Variations

To awaken any sleeping senses, try starting with light, repeated tapping of the tip of your tongue on the head of her clit. Her clit will be very sensitive when you first touch it, so go softly. Don't pull back the clitoral hood because that will deliver way too much stimulation, and might even hurt. "I like my clit played with gently," says Tawny. "I only like it rougher after I am turned on, that's when I want someone to suck on it." There are licks, cat laps, and back-and-forth or up-and-down flicks. All of these can be done with the tip, or with the smoother and softer flat area of your tongue, and all produce different sensations. Some women prefer their guys to go in a circular motion on their clit, and we even heard a story about one guy, an industrious student of sex, who used to trace the letters of the alphabet. As you feel her clit get harder, apply a little more pressure.

Your tongue can also be a tool of penetration. Try rolling it into a cylinder and moving you head so that your tongue slides in and out of her vagina or anus. The roughness of your tongue on the sensitive opening and walls of her vagina will be very stimulating, and the penetration will be a great warm-up to things that may come later. Sunrise adores this technique, after being properly warmed up, of course: "At first I like the tongue really soft and slow, with his tongue focused on my clit. Then, as I get more turned on, I like a swipe from my crotch up to my clit. Then I like the tongue inside. Start off slow and then get more aggressive."

It's extremely helpful for a woman to give her partner some idea of what she likes and doesn't like. A soft "umm, that feels great," or "yes, keep it right on there," is all she needs to convey to let him know he's doing okay. If she wants him to change motions or pressure, she might say "ooh, a little softer" or "gently now" if he's going too hard or fast, or "faster, harder" or "don't stop" if she's getting close to orgasm.

But guys should also realize that a woman may not know exactly what she likes, especially if she's never felt a certain sensation before. She may not be able to give you detailed directions because, let's face it, she's not really in a position to see what's going on down there. Guys should also understand that if a woman reaches down to add her own hands into the mix, they shouldn't feel offended. It doesn't mean you're doing a lousy job; it means she wants to supplement your licks with her own touch for maximum pleasure. But whatever you do, it's probably going to feel great because everything will get really wet and hot. So experiment.

Advanced Techniques

❝ I'm not into hours of foreplay, but I do like fifteen to twenty minutes. I like oral sex, followed by a vibrator. ❞

—Mercedez

As she becomes more aroused, your partner will most likely want you to stop working every angle possible and focus on her clitoris. At that point, she may also want more intense stimulation (but remember, no rule applies to all women; when in doubt, ask!). Now may be the time to try sucking on her clitoris.

Jenna explains her preferred technique: "My partner has this certain thing with me, I call it 'the suck and click.' I'm not exactly sure how he does it, but he sucks my clit in and flicks it at the same time. Three minutes of that and it's all over with! We've been together for four and a half years, so he knows exactly what it takes." To replicate Jenna's "suck and click" technique, with your mouth directly over the clit, you can suck it into your mouth and tweak it with your tongue at the same time. You can practice this without a partner—stick your tongue out through your lips. Now as you pull it back into your mouth, suck at the same time. You'll hear a little "pop." That's the "click" part. When you try it on her, the clit will be in the mix as well, just above your tongue. Try it to see if she likes it. Some women only like this near the end, and others, who have a very sensitive clit, find it's too much. Mercedez is one of them. "I don't like my clit sucked at all. It just doesn't feel good. When a girl did it to me, it was too intense, it almost hurt."

To get a good view of some suck-and-click action, check out *Where the Boys Aren't 15*. There's a hot scene between Kira and Dasha in which Kira does some doubling up, moving both her tongue and head backward and forward, along with some awesome clit sucking. At one point, Dasha puts her legs in the air in a V as Kira darts her tongue in and out of Dasha's ass, while sucking her clit at the same time. In the same film, there's a steamy-hot all-girl threesome with Briana in a bathroom during which you'll see and hear, "Suck it! Eat that pussy."

Other exciting advanced techniques can be seen in *Obsession*— one sizzling-hot film. In this gem, you'll see the technique of using saliva to keep things wet, the excitement of hearing lots of slurping noises, licking and flicking with a pierced tongue, and the use of a vibrator combined with oral sex.

Adding Hands

Don't forget to make use of your supporting cast, especially your hands. Obviously, you can spread your partner's thighs apart and hold your hands there for a while. You can place both your palms right under her bottom and dive in like you were eating a delicious watermelon. You can use the thumb and index finger of one hand to keep her lips spread for your mouth. You can also do this by making a "V for victory" sign with your forefinger and middle finger while your tongue goes between them. And, you can keep things open by rhythmically using your thumbs to open and hold her labia. Two more tips: Most women really like their partner to put the fingers of one hand on their pubic mound and stretch the skin back toward the stomach. Others like their partners to rub the mound rapidly while they lick. This is a very sexy gesture, and one that really focuses sensation on the clit.

Don't forget that your hands are free to roam about the other deliciously hungry areas of her body. Play with her breasts, stroke her thighs, tweak her nipples, squeeze her ass, do whatever feels right. You should also make eye contact with her, and take a breather every once in a while and tell her how much you are enjoying yourself. If you get tired (and most men do), try changing positions to alleviate neck or jaw stress or alternate between stimulating her with your mouth and your hand.

You can also use a free hand to slip a finger or two inside her.

Many women love the sensation of penetration while being licked, while others like to stay focused on their clit. Another movement your woman might like is cunnilingus alternating with clit tapping. We'll cover the finer points of manual penetration and other hand actions in the Chapter 7, but if you want plenty of combined hand and oral action, a great film to see is *Swoosh*. There's some great stuff happening in the beginning of the film out by the swimming pool, as well as some hot girl-on-girl jailhouse scenes.

Rhythm Methods

❝❝ **It's important to keep steady rhythm, because if you break the rhythm, you have to start all over. Once you find that certain thing that drives her wild, stick with it, and don't stop until she comes.** ❞❞

—Jenna

Jenna's right, once a woman is really turned on, rhythm and consistency are everything. After you find that perfect motion of your tongue and the amount of pressure that makes her gasp, by all means, stick with it! The more you stay focused on your technique, the hotter she will get, and she may even have an orgasm. It's pretty safe to say that you should go slower to entice her in the beginning, and keep up a steady rhythm as she gets close to coming. Another good film in which to observe rhythm is *The Vision,* where Helen of Troy and her guy have an extended session. And, just like men, some women like their partner to keep a tongue on their clit after they've come, while others find that their clit is much too sensitive. Some women even like their partner to start up the motion again after a few seconds as they head toward orgasm number two, three, four, or more. (We'll discuss more about multiple orgasms in Chapter 11.)

Team Vivid varies on how much time you should spend down under. Dasha prefers a brief cunnilingus foray: "I guess it depends on how you do it. I do like it, but just a little bit of it, because it gets me too excited, and I'm just like 'come on, let's do it right now!' I don't go for a half hour of it." Kira says, "I like oral sex, but not for very long. Get me going, then I want something else." Sometimes, it just depends on her mood: "There are days when I want romance and lots of foreplay. But there are also times when I am not your typical girl, especially when I haven't had sex for a while. I want to cut to the chase," she adds.

Bobby believes in the opposite philosophy: "This is advice my uncle gave me: spend a good hour licking her pussy and you can't go wrong. For most women, it's a surefire way to give her an orgasm." Jenna agrees that persistence and stamina are key: "Sometimes I'll do it on purpose and try not to come for like forty-five minutes. I can hear him gasping for air, but he hangs in there, and that's the sign of a very good man." Alternatively, Kira likes oral sex after her orgasm: "I like it afterward, especially if the sex has been superintense because it's more soothing than anything. If the sex has been so intense, you're throbbing down there. Just take it slow, just barely licking, and that's great. I'm so happy I found a man who's willing to do things after the orgasm." Whichever way you and your partner prefer it, remember to have fun while you are at it.

Up Close & Personal
★ Mercedez ★

The former Miss Nude Universe and Exotic Dancer Entertainer of the Year (2002), Mercedez dances in the premiere gentlemen's clubs in the country three weeks out of every month. The jump into movies seemed like a logical one, since she felt she had reached the pinnacle of success in the dancing world.

The climb through the ranks of exotic dancers has

been a sexual education for Mercedez. "I learned to enjoy sex from stripping. Before I started dancing, sex wasn't that great at all. I wasn't open to different positions. But if you watch a house dancer give a table dance, you'll see her try different positions that guys' wives won't do. It's a more open attitude toward sex, and dancing opened that up for me." In fact, Mercedez says that when she is dancing, one of her favorite sexy hot spots for having sex is the dressing room.

A few weeks after Mercedez was chosen as the Miss Nude Universe 2003, she decided to shoot her first-ever adult feature. The voluptuous, five-foot six-and-a-half-inch brunette from Corpus Christi, Texas, was signed immediately as a Vivid Girl, the top rung among adult film actresses.

Since she began appearing in adult movies, Mercedez has learned a lot from other performers in the industry. She believes adult movies have a lot to teach people, and she thinks consumers of porn make better lovers. "You know the guys who are going to be the worst in bed are the ones who have perfect hair and perfect tans. They are young and think they are so hot, but you know they are inexperienced. I like to look at them, but I think to myself, 'He's just going to piss me off in bed.' I'd much rather go with a regular guy. Just a regular guy, especially one who says, 'I watch porn all the time; I watch the Playboy Channel.' Those are the guys I want to take home. You know they will be open to trying stuff."

Mercedez's favorite thing to try with new fellas is playing with toys. "Toys are my favorite thing, and I don't like guys who aren't open to that. Some guys are intimidated by toys." To introduce toys into their sex, Mercedez usually asked, "Do you want to do something fun? I'll bring out a vibrator and show him how to use it. Once we get that going, I'd bring out a dildo and let him use that on me."

Her personal collection includes about twenty different vibrators. "I have the one with the butterfly, the flower, one that glows in the dark. And I have a lot of dildos, too." When it comes to dildos Mercedez has tried many kinds. "I prefer the jelly kind. The ones that are realistic-looking CyberSkin pick up fuzz and carpet fiber too easily, and in the heat of the moment you don't want to be fumbling trying to get it into the box to keep it off the carpet when you're in the middle of having sex. You have to have some kind of special powder to clean them and that's a pain."

She mixes the toys in with other erotic actions. "With the vibrator I like to put it on my clit while he is down there doing oral. And it's nice to have it on there while I am doing him, too. And if I am going to have any kind of anal, I have to have a vibrator to help me relax and make the penetration feel good at the beginning. And when it comes to the dildo, I like him to grab it with both hands and fuck me with it. I am not into soft sex. I like hard penetration and that way I'm always satisfied."

Mercedez says her favorite sex scene was with Chris Cannon in the movie *Women in Uniform*. "Chris is professional, he's great at his job. He's good at oral sex—not all porn stars are!" She's also looking forward to trying two guys on film. "Two guys sounds interesting to me, just because watching it turns me on, so I think doing it will be fun, too. I've never done a threesome with a guy and a girl either, so I'm excited to give that a try on film. I look forward to role-playing, being in the movies, and trying on different roles." She also says, "I'm open to sharing everything. I don't think I'm too much of a 'save that for home' type. If I've done it with my husband, it's okay to do it on film.

Mercedez describes herself as "everything a Scorpio is said to be." Despite her amazing physique, she loves bubble baths, body lotions, sexy perfumes, and skimpy nighties. "I am a girlie girl, but I am also a fitness fanatic and my favorite reading is magazines like *Muscle, Muscular Development,* and *Muscle & Fitness.*" She's an ideal date, who likes nothing more than to settle down in front of the VCR to watch horror movies like *Night Breed* or *Pumpkin Head,* maybe an *Austin Powers* comedy, or something with Sylvester Stallone or Vin Diesel. She loves Thai food, but mostly she's a health-food junkie. She also hasn't lost all of her rural Lone Star tastes. "I am a true truck girl. I like Ford F-350s and Hummers." And what's this sexy brunette's favorite music? "I guess I am stuck in the eighties as far as music goes, since the Cult is my favorite group and I love Ian Astbury." She likes anything by Prince and Sade for music to have sex to.

In addition to her honor as Miss Nude Universe 2003, Mercedez was chosen as Miss Nude North America and Miss Nude International 2001 and 2002. She also received the 2002–2003 Golden G-String Award and was acclaimed as Miss Nude World's Hardest Body. Mercedez has appeared on the cover and in pictorials in *Penthouse, Gent* magazine, *Muscular Development, Exotic Dancers Annual 2002 Directory, Club International* Leg Action, *Hustler* Busty

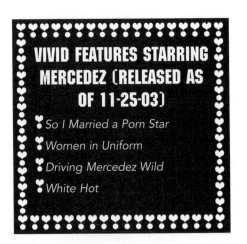

VIVID FEATURES STARRING MERCEDEZ (RELEASED AS OF 11-25-03)

❣ *So I Married a Porn Star*

❣ *Women in Uniform*

❣ *Driving Mercedez Wild*

❣ *White Hot*

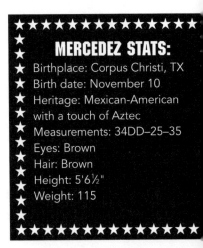

MERCEDEZ STATS:

★ Birthplace: Corpus Christi, TX
★ Birth date: November 10
★ Heritage: Mexican-American
★ with a touch of Aztec
★ Measurements: 34DD–25–35
★ Eyes: Brown
★ Hair: Brown
★ Height: 5'6½"
★ Weight: 115

Beauties, *Swanks* Open Legs and Lace, *Swanks* Leg Action, *Gallery* magazine, *Fox* magazine, and *Leg Tease.* Mercedez has also appeared on *The Jenny Jones Show,* and was a Sin Avisio video girl, a Budweiser calendar girl, an Elegant Moments model, and a Latin Video girl. Olé!

6
going down (on him)

Fantasy File:

He lies back on the low bed covered in soft satiny sheets. He'd always found Asian women especially attractive, drawn to their jet-black hair and dark brown eyes. And now, a fantasy fulfilled. To each side of him: a young, beautiful woman whose sole aim at the moment is to please him. Each has long, dark hair that trails over the shoulders toward her stomach. The woman in red leans across his chest and massages his shoulders and chest. As she pulls away, she licks and kisses those same spots. The woman in blue gently tweaks his nipple—he didn't think he would like that, but to his surprise, he does—as she glides down his stomach toward his cock. She looks into his eyes—a deep and penetrating stare—before putting his penis into her mouth. She stretches her body down the length of his leg, gently rubbing her pussy against his thigh. She circles the head of his dick with her tongue, then takes it all in at once. With a pent-up sexual energy, she slides his dick quickly in and out of her mouth while pumping at the shaft with her hand.

He feels the second girl kissing and licking his belly now. He throws his head back and closes his eyes as he begins to feel two warm sensuous mouths near his penis. The girl in blue moves down to his balls as the girl in red takes over on his shaft. The touch of her lips feels slightly different; she sucks just on the head as she glides her hand up and down the shaft. The girl in blue takes his balls in her mouth as she tugs slightly at the base. The pleasure of having his balls and cock sucked at the same time sends shock waves through his groin. After a moment, he can't tell which girl is working on which part as he loses himself in the sheer excitement of it all.

As the girl in red continues sucking, he massages her upturned buttock and then glides his finger past the moist lips of her vagina. The girls now take turns sucking his dick, passing it back and forth from one mouth to the other. In between, the girl in blue continues to tug and lick his balls. He becomes even more excited as he watches their mouths come together on his shaft and they kiss each other. As their heads move up and down, their hair gently tickles his inner thighs. Wanting more, he probes his fingers deeper into the girl's pussy.

The girls are now side by side on their hands on knees in front of him. He enters the first girl from behind. She backs into him to take in the full length of his hard cock. He pulls out, then rubs his dick up and down over her clitoris, which shocks her with delight. He reenters her and thrusts back and forth; each time he pulls back so far that the ridge of his dick emerges from inside. With renewed hunger, she pulls his whole penis back inside with her vaginal muscles, filling her up with his fat, hard cock. He moves to the second girl and enters her from behind. The first girl massages the other's back and thighs. When she delivers a firm smack to the other's buttock, he feels a slight tensing in her muscles, which excites him even more.

"Yes, yes," she moans with pleasure, her head resting on a pillow while her rear extends upward for his continued thrusting. He likes hearing her tell him what she wants, and he fucks her with added fervor. As he's doing this, the first girl kisses the second on her neck and shoulders, massages her back and breasts, tugging on her erect nipples. The second girl moans and sighs with pleasure as all her erogenous zones are stimulated at once.

The girls turn on their backs, and he continues fucking them: first one and then the other. Their collective pleasure amplifies as each moves closer and closer to climax. As he fucks the girl in red, he watches the girl in blue massage her own clitoris and breasts. The girls' moans are matched by his own sighs and heavy breathing caused by the force of his exertions. "Yes, yes," the girls shout, wanting still more. With each push, he feels his dick getting bigger and more sensitive. Finally, unable to fuck anymore, he pulls out, stands up, and shoots his huge load across the bed onto the two girls. It streams out of him as he finishes himself off with his hand. He shudders with each small shot of semen, until there is none left. Still shaking, he leans down and kisses the girls on the lips, a long slow kiss after an exhausting and energetic round of sex.

★★ *from* Bangkok Nights,
directed by Toni English

❝ The thing I look forward to doing the most would have to be blow jobs. I mean, come on. I think a lot of girls, especially my friends, look forward to doing it because it's the one way a girl can really go and blow a guy's mind. And if you take the initiative, guys can tell you really enjoy it. ❞

—Jenna

Since we've never met a man who'd turn down a blow job, working on your oral expertise is one of the best ways to enhance your sexual repertoire. Briana, Sunrise, Savanna, and Jenna all say they consider blow jobs their specialty, and they cite BJs as the thing they love most to do. The blow job is, of course, a staple in just about every sex scene in every adult film ever made. The sight of a woman's face and lips juxtaposed with an erect penis is a striking and erotic image, one that most men dream of daily. The blow job can stand alone, or be incorporated into a longer scene. Sunrise favors a "BJ only" scenario when she is too tired for more. "If I am tired, it doesn't always have to be about intercourse. I give my man a full-body massage and a blow job, and we both go to sleep happy," she says. Alternatively, oral sex can be a first course leading into something more. The more stimulation before the orgasm, the bigger that orgasm will be. Willingness, a little initiative, and some enthusiasm will do wonders for your BJ technique.

Just Breathe

As with other erotic acts, a little teasing is in order before getting down to business. As you move your head down toward his groin, he'll expect you to start sucking right away. Instead, make him wait a bit and you'll have his full attention. The Vivid Girls have found that a few sexy words can do wonders to increase his excitement. Before going down on him, tell him how sexy he is, what you want to do to him, or how much he turns you on. Before going any further, open your mouth and exhale a slow warm breath over his cock and balls. Then move your head up and down the shaft without touching him to build up his anticipation even more.

Place the lips over the head of his penis, and then suck it into your mouth. Be sure to have some saliva in your mouth to help it lubricate him as it slides in. Kira advises: "Make it wet, use lots of spit." More important, she recommends making eye contact while going down on a guy. "People tell me I have a hunger in my eyes and it turns them on. It's important to express how much you love what you're doing," she adds. The mental connection is also noted by Bobby. "Some guys are just happy that a girl will do it at all, but I guess I've developed higher standards," he says. "I get off easy, so it's not so much what you do as how much love and enthusiasm you put into it." And the best way to show this, of course, is through some Kira-like eye contact.

Once the head of his penis is in your mouth, use your tongue to get at the sensitive areas. The most sensitive spot of all is that little V-shaped spot just under the ridge of the head (the area that will be facing you if it's standing straight up). The light roughness of your tongue will feel good as you move it from side to side across the head or in a circle just underneath there. If you have a pierced tongue, all the better. Briana says, "I swirl my tongue around the head a lot. I also have my tongue pierced and he can really feel that."

Grease the Pole

To create a smooth motion with your mouth, you need to make it slick. "Spit is the best lube for a blow job, and lots of it," states Jenna. "The further down your throat you can get it, the better your spit is," she adds helpfully. If your spit can't cut it, you can use an added lubricant. Flavored lubes are made specifically for oral sex, so you might want to pick one up on your next visit to the toy store. Another Vivid Girl tip: keep your tongue on top of your bottom teeth, or purse your lips to cover your teeth, to avoid any painful scraping as you move up and down. "No teeth at all," exclaims Justin plainly, "keep your teeth off the cock." There you have it.

In terms of style, there are a couple of different approaches. Savanna likes a slow, multitasking approach. "I don't go too fast at first. Suck his cock a little; look into his eyes while you're doing it. And don't forget the other parts of his body: his nipples, his neck. You might forget to go there, but it can be really exciting for a guy and it keeps him aroused." If the cock in question is especially wide (as is often the case on a film shoot), it may be difficult to get your mouth around it. Moistening your lips with saliva and tucking them over your teeth will make it easier. You can also glide your lips and tongue up and down the outside of the shaft.

Watch and Learn!

In *The Vision,* two bored dot-com types hire two girls to come to their house. Blond beauty Dasha gives some pretty great head in the beginning scene. First, she gets right down to business and takes as much of the guy's huge cock in her mouth as she can. She uses her right hand to press down at the base of the penis, which keeps his penis standing straight up and prevents it from flopping around during her oral ministrations. She licks up and down the sides to keep it slick, then she delivers a little oral excitement to his balls, which are also pretty hefty. Too big to fit into her mouth all at once, Dasha gently takes one ball in her mouth at a time and lightly sucks on it. Starting at the very base of his balls, she also licks all the way up and over them toward his shaft. Another little trick she performs—one we've never seen before—is that she spits on her nipple, rubs the head of his dick on it, then flicks his dick on her breast. All in all, a major hot move. Her female costar has some good BJ moves, too, as she blows the other dot-commer on the other side of the room. He stands while she kneels before him. In between licking and sucking his dick, she also nuzzles her face in his balls and lightly licks them. She's also a pro at the whole eye-contact thing, and she looks up at him alluringly throughout the blow job. Another little move she excels at is incorporating her hand into action. Wrapping her whole hand around his dick, she moves up and down in sync with her mouth, stimulating his whole rod at once.

That last move is one that many of the Vivid Girls recommend, particularly if your partner is well endowed. Justin puts it this way: "As you move your lips up and down the shaft, use your hand to make the same motion. Don't be lazy! Make it enjoyable and get off on getting the guy off." Mercedez adds: "I like to suck on the head and work the rest with my hand. I have a bad gag reflex, so I've learned to work it good with my hands. I can also make up for it with a lot of tongue. I'll run my tongue all the way down to the balls, then back up to the top, where I lick the whole head. While I do that I move my hands up and down, too."

Practice Makes Perfect

❝❝ I learned how to give head on a banana, I learned how to deep-throat bananas without breaking them, and I learned how to deep-throat with no gag reflex. I think I was naturally good at it. ❞❞

—*Sunrise*

Many women are concerned about the gag reflex when giving head. It varies by individual; some women are very sensitive to it, while others hardly gag at all. "I have no gag reflex, so I can naturally deep-throat," says Briana. "I never knew I had this specialty until I was in the business and had to work with some very well-endowed men." Not all women are as lucky as Briana, and it's a perfectly natural reaction for a person to gag when something touches certain areas near the back of the mouth and throat. Often, the physical reaction is accompanied by a psychological anticipation of it, which makes gagging almost inevitable. The good news is that you can learn to suppress this natural reflex. Going slowly, the Girls advise, make a swallowing motion with your throat as the penis hits the back of your mouth. They say it's similar to the move you make when trying to clear your ears when they are stuffed up. With practice, your timing will improve and eventually come naturally. Another tip is to try different angles of insertion to see which works best for you. Savanna admits, "I try to stick it far down my throat, but I'm not that good at it. Every once in a while, though, you get the angle just right."

Most of the girls agree that the psychological component of gagging is as intense as the physical one. "Lots of women are nervous about giving head, afraid of gagging, or of doing it wrong," says Sunrise. "Relax the back of your throat, enjoy it, and get into it." Relaxation is key to overcoming any anxiety you have about oral sex. Mercedez got over her gag reflex by practicing a lot with her partner. "I think it's all in my mind," she says. "You just have to let yourself relax, and put the worry of gagging out of your mind." Similarly, Tawny also had a bad gag reflex. "Eventually, I learned to open the back of my throat. If you practice, you can get it. Practice makes perfect," she says brightly.

In *Filthy Rich,* one of the three evil daughters vying for Daddy's money goes down on the family lawyer in a big way. While he sits on an overstuffed sofa she kneels on the floor in front of him and delivers the blow job of a lifetime. Her special recipe involves taking just the tip of the penis into her mouth, making a tight seal around it with her lips and then popping it out. While sucking on the head, she also does a great two handed palm twist on the shaft that really gets him going.

Hands-on

For those who are still a little shy about giving a good blow job, remember that using you hand is not "cheating." Jenna says, "Slow, rhythmic blow jobs are awesome. If you rush too much it's not as good. He may come faster, but the orgasm isn't as good." She recommends using your hand and mouth at the same time. "That way," she adds, "if your mouth gets tired, you can let your hand take over while you recover a little." To go the extra mile, try Dasha's two-hand tunnel-of-love move. "Wrap both hands around the penis, slide up and down, and go over it at the same time with your mouth. It makes him feel like he's inside, because you create this hole with a soft end. Sometimes I like to twist my head so it adds more stimulation, corkscrewing up and down, while twisting at the same time." For a demo of the head twist, check out Dasha and the professor in *Student Body.*

One of the most fabled oral sex positions is, of course, the 69. In *Jenna Loves Rocco,* there is a great scene on a round bed where the two stars do an extended 69. He lies flat on his back while she sits on his face and gives him head. This 69-style position is great for the woman giving head because it changes the angle of entry completely, and many women feel more comfortable coming at the penis from above rather than below. It works especially well if the guy's penis curves upward, as many do. In this scene, she takes all of his huge rod in her mouth, has both hands free to accompany her, and has the added bonus of getting head from him at the same time.

> ❝ **Don't forget the balls. I always touch the balls somehow, stroking them, holding them, licking them.** ❞
>
> —Kira

Cutting the balls in on the action is another great way to bump up your BJ to a new level. The key is to start gently and see how your guy likes it. Because their balls are so sensitive, many guys are a little apprehensive when you first touch them. So start slowly, then explore a few different sensations to see what works best for him. For starters, as you're pumping your mouth up and down on his shaft, use one of your free hands on the balls. Some men enjoy the sensation of their balls being petted in time with your mouth motions. Others like a bit of tickling or stroking with your fingertips or light gentle teasing with the fingernails. Still others like a gentle tug downward on the whole sac. Savanna recommends being up front about ball play and asking flat out. "I always ask because I find that men are very particular about their balls. I like to lick them, put them in to my mouth slowly, and stroke him at the same time. Sometimes, I drag my fingernails across them, and that makes some guys come," she says. Another trick is to give your mouth a break by relaxing your jaw, then sliding your tongue and mouth over his balls. Tawny says: "I like to suck on his balls as I play with his cock. It's a total tease to take your mouth off his dick and put it elsewhere."

Watch and Learn!

In *Intimate Journey,* a man's girlfriend catches him fooling around with another girl and then joins in the action. Later in the film, three couples get it on in the backyard, all while watching one another. There's some great oral action by one couple. The woman kneels in front of the guy to give him a BJ, but also does a little technique known as "teabagging." This handy method is where you take both balls into

BJ CHEAT SHEET

1. Open wide.
2. Relax your throat muscles.
3. Keep it wet.
4. Try the two-hand twist
5. Relax some more.
6. Take it all in at once.
7. Explore nearby regions.
8. Tell him how much you like it.

your mouth as Tawny recommends above. With the balls in your mouth, you gently tug the whole package down slightly, sort of like dipping a tea bag in a cup of hot water. In the film, she licks all around his thighs and groin, teabags him, and "pets" his balls, too.

In *Student Body,* one of the girls from the Tri Twat sorority vies for the BJ crown. She gets it on with two football players at the same time. As one guy bangs her from behind, she delivers some hot oral action to another guy in front. She puts his penis in her mouth, then takes little breathers in between while using her hand. She adds a nice little topspin to her hand strokes and keeps him well lubricated with her saliva. She also licks up and down his entire shaft and massages his balls when her mouth is full, and does it all with a smile on her face. Needless to say, she wins the crown: a black hat with a giant dildo on top, which she wears proudly after the guys bestow it upon her.

If you're feeling even more adventurous, you might want to explore another area down there that's sure to please: his rear end. Some guys can still be a bit touchy about anal stimulation, afraid they might come off as gay. But these days, with hot moves available for viewing twenty-four hours a day, a lot of guys have quickly shed that inhibition. Start with some preliminary strokes with your fingertips and then gently go inside just a little. If he seems to like it, then lube up your finger and move it in and out very slowly. If your mouth is down there, then lick the area that extends from his balls to his ass, going all the way up the crack between his cheeks. Once you try this, few guys will tell you to stop. Since you're in the neighborhood, try licking the rim of his asshole. Justin says: "Don't be afraid to eat ass. If you're going to to eat the guy's penis, then why not keep going." You can check out more tips on anal action in "Bend Over Babes and Boys" (Chapter 10).

❝ ❝ **Every guy likes a sloppy blow job, but what turns a guy on even more is basically telling him how much you want to 'worship' it, how big it is, how much you love his balls, and how much of a turn-on it is to feel them slapping against you. No matter what, after this, he's got a big head on it.** ❞ ❞

—Kira

★ Bobby Vitale ★
Up Close & Personal

Bobby Vitale didn't expect to end up in adult movies, but a failed relationship was the first step for him: "I was going out with this girl for some time, and then it went south on us. She started seeing another guy, and she was trying to make me jealous. She told me they had a great sex life and they watched the Playboy Channel together a lot."

Vitale ran a very successful car-detailing business, and one of his clients was a porn producer. Vitale approached him and asked if he could perform in an adult movie. He admits his motivation was revenge: "I wanted to be in a film just to make this woman jealous. I knew she would eventually see me on television. Maybe three or six months later, I wanted to reconcile with her. She told me that her mother saw me on the Playboy Channel, and we wouldn't be getting back together anytime soon. I know that I didn't get into the adult industry in the usual way. I got into it as a novelty, but I realized it was more lucrative (and more fun) than the auto detailing business." So, he joined the adult industry full-time, and has since made over two hundred movies.

Bobby was encouraged by other men in the industry. Early on, he was mentored by stars like Ron Jeremy and Peter North, who gave him advice along the way: "I worked with Ron Jeremy on some films that he directed. He's one of the funniest guys in the business, but also one of the best. I also really respect Rocco Siffredi. Without men like these guys coming before, not only me, but also the new guys after me, would be nowhere. Male performers TT Boy and Peter North really mentored me. Peter gave me some great pep talks. I was so nervous at first. TT Boy was in my first movie, so he was on the set, but he doesn't hang out and talk with people much. He's very low-key. Working with him, I felt like I was working next to John Wayne. I was just starstruck, and he pulled me aside, told me, 'Whatever the situation, you're going to have chemistry with some people, and with some, you're not. You have to tap into your fantasies, and use them to make your performance better.' He compared it to an athlete who uses visualization. Now I tell the new guys the same things—that you have to respect your 'godfathers.' Without them and the guys before them, you'd be nowhere. Rocco Siffredi, Mark Davis, Tom Byron, Ron Jeremy—I respect all those guys."

Advice from other performers led him to explore what turned him on. "Getting into the business has helped me get in touch with my fantasies. I like to mix romance and being naughty, and go from one to the other—drag her into the bathroom and do some kinky stuff in there, then take her back to the bed and make her feel like a princess. I can be pretty aggressive, but I do it in a loving way. Sometimes, I think about taking a really pretty girl to a real dirty place, like in an alley by a dumpster or in the car, because you know no one else has taken her there. And I like her to look into my eyes during sex, because I want her to know who's making love to her. Ultimately, I like to make a girl feel like she's been well satisfied, especially if she's with someone else, she'll think of me."

Bobby has been in an on-again, off-again relationship with Vivid Girl Briana Banks for several years. Even though they are both adult performers, they still have feelings of jealousy, so they set certain ground rules. "Briana and I have a great relationship. I know everybody she works with, they are my peers or the guys who taught me, and I respect them. I am never on the same set with her when she is performing with someone else, and she does the same for me. Once, I was doing a scene with another woman for Club Jenna, and Briana came to the set, and I got a "flat tire." My heart just dropped to my knees like I was cheating. I think it's normal for us to get a little jealous, and we wouldn't be human if we didn't have those feelings. We get through it because we are honest with each other."

Beside the fact that they were together, Bobby loves working with her. "I have been with Briana for a long time, but every time I've worked with her, I was so turned on. I saw every side of her, her bad days and good, and I had sex with her whenever I wanted. But still, I had so much energy and passion for her on film—I could go through three condoms—that was something special." He has some advice for other couples: "You have to please your girl first. For guys, it gets old after a while, so I say just keep switching it up. Get a nice suite at a hotel, stock it with champagne and chocolate-dipped strawberries, and make it an evening to remember."

Bobby believes that porn can be a positive part of

people's lives. "We're in the happiness business. People, whether they are single or in a relationship, watch us and we give them pleasure."

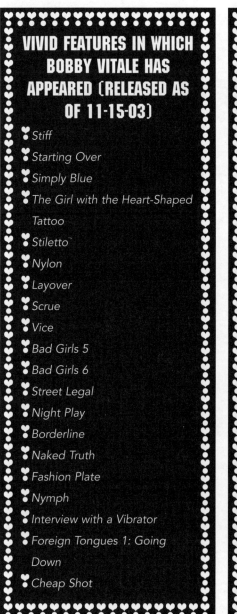

VIVID FEATURES IN WHICH BOBBY VITALE HAS APPEARED (RELEASED AS OF 11-15-03)

- Stiff
- Starting Over
- Simply Blue
- The Girl with the Heart-Shaped Tattoo
- Stiletto
- Nylon
- Layover
- Scrue
- Vice
- Bad Girls 5
- Bad Girls 6
- Street Legal
- Night Play
- Borderline
- Naked Truth
- Fashion Plate
- Nymph
- Interview with a Vibrator
- Foreign Tongues 1: Going Down
- Cheap Shot
- Illicit Entry
- Jenteal Loves Rocco
- Party House
- Chasey Loves Rocco
- Ghost Town
- Body Language
- Sex Gallery
- Pleasureland
- Manic Behavior
- Introducing Alexis
- Suggestive Behavior
- The End
- Head to Head
- Interview with a Milkman
- This Year's Model
- Lethal Affairs
- ECU: Janine
- Hard Feelings
- I Want It All
- Rebel Cheerleader
- Viewpoint
- Born Bad
- Sweet Revenge
- Rolling Thunder
- Photoplay
- Heat

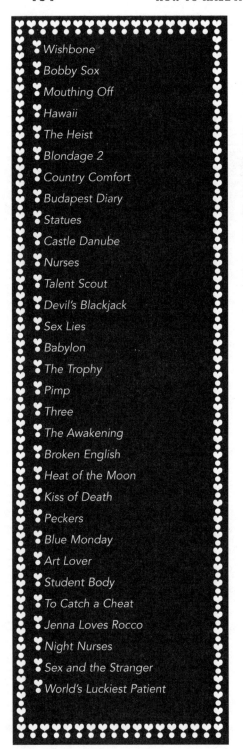

- Wishbone
- Bobby Sox
- Mouthing Off
- Hawaii
- The Heist
- Blondage 2
- Country Comfort
- Budapest Diary
- Statues
- Castle Danube
- Nurses
- Talent Scout
- Devil's Blackjack
- Sex Lies
- Babylon
- The Trophy
- Pimp
- Three
- The Awakening
- Broken English
- Heat of the Moon
- Kiss of Death
- Peckers
- Blue Monday
- Art Lover
- Student Body
- To Catch a Cheat
- Jenna Loves Rocco
- Night Nurses
- Sex and the Stranger
- World's Luckiest Patient

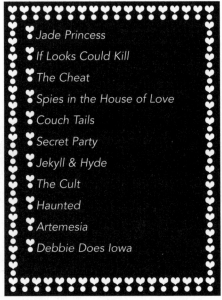

- Jade Princess
- If Looks Could Kill
- The Cheat
- Spies in the House of Love
- Couch Tails
- Secret Party
- Jekyll & Hyde
- The Cult
- Haunted
- Artemesia
- Debbie Does Iowa

7
give that lovely lady a hand

Fantasy File:

The customer stands near her car while the mechanic lies flat on her back, working beneath the vehicle. As the customer waits for her car, she wears a tiny white tank top and a pair of really high cutoff jeans that show off plenty of her tight, toned ass and the tattoo on the back of her long, shapely leg. The mechanic slides out from under the car. Even in her jeans and black work boots, her voluptuous breasts stand out underneath her skimpy shirt. She motions for the customer to tell her about the problem. In Tony's All-Girl Garage, they fix lots of things besides cars and pickup trucks.

"Sometimes when I'm driving, I can't even hear the music," the sexy customer says in a deep Southern drawl. My car makes such a noise; I don't know what it is."

"What else can you tell me?" asks the mechanic, eyeing her up and down.

"When I'm trying to put on my makeup in the rearview mirror, it pulls to the side; to the right a little bit." And pausing for only a moment, she adds, "What do you see?"

The mechanic reaches up to stroke the customer's leg. "It's all good," she says as her hand moves higher, settling on the ass of the magnificent stranger whose car just happened to find its way to this unique garage.

As the hand touches her skin, a bolt of electricity shoots through the customer's body. She eyes the mechanic momentarily, puts one leg up on the car bumper, then turns her ass toward the seductive laborer. Within seconds, their clothes are off and strewn around the dirty concrete floor of the garage. The mechanic puts one hand on each of the girl's pussy lips, spreads them as wide as she can, and then mashes her sweaty face into their soft, fragrant wetness. The customer, looking for immediate satisfaction, rapidly taps her own clit while the mechanic inserts a finger inside the customer's quivering cunt, drilling in and out of the hot sticky slit, turning and twisting her finger as if she were screwing in a bolt.

"Yeah, fuck me," says the customer. "Yeah, yeah, oh yeah."

The mechanic turns her tongue to the girl's asshole, then changes the deliberate twist-and-screw motion of her finger into rapid sideways strokes. Soon after her sweet release, the tables turn, and the customer services the mechanic.

Their bodies glisten in the Southern heat as they change places. The customer unzips the worker's jeans, pulls them off, and licks the soft flesh of her ass cheeks. Turning her over once more, she gently fondles the mechanic's breasts, and then heads lower, first inserting one curved finger to find her G-spot, then using two or three. At the same time, the handy mechanic presses firmly on her own pubic mound, brushing her fingers over her now erect clit. The blonde swings her long hair back from her face. Revealing she's no ingenue when it comes to this type of servicing, the customer stretches wide the mechanic's pussy lips, then darts her tongue in and out to keep it lubed up. Using the flat parts of her fingers on the mechanic's clit knob, first she brushes lightly, then rubs in a circle until the walls of the garage echo with cries of pleasure.

Changing places once again, the comely customer

leans back, opens her legs wide, and lifts her knees up behind her ears. The mechanic uses her masterful hands and tongue skillfully, then surprises the customer by rubbing her own nipple on the blonde's aching clit. The girl is insatiable, screaming for more.

Once again, the mechanic darts her tongue in and out of the girl's puckered ass opening, stopping only long enough to rub her clit rapidly from side to side. As she nibbles on the girl's cunt lips, the customer—always hungry for more—reaches down to rub her own clit in a wild frenzy.

"Here I come," she cries. "Yeah, yeah, yeah, yeah."

★★ *from Where the Boys Aren't 15,*
directed by Chi Chi LaRue

Tips for Men on Hand Jobs for Her

❝ **I like when a guy is inventive with his hands.** ❞

—*Jenna*

In Chapter 5, we sang the praises of oral stimulation, but your tongue is not your only tool to make a woman purr. You can continue the work your mouth does to stimulate her clitoris with a helping hand— your own. Like oral sex, manual stimulation of her vagina, clitoris, and, if she's into it, her anus is a great way to get her turned on. You can use your hands to work your way up to intercourse, or penetration with a dildo; or use them as an exciting addition to intercourse. Fingers make great stimulation tools: they're agile, flexible, and connected to your brain. Not only can you create lots of different sensations with those digits, but you can feel how her body responds to certain kinds of stimulation. Make sure your nails are clean, short, and well filed—you want them to feel smooth and sexy as they explore her. Fingers not only feel good, but they also help warm her up for bigger things to come. Try these techniques, and she may never look at your hands the same way again.

Teasing and Touching

There is a lot of fun to be had South of the Border, so let's take it one step at a time, beginning with external stimulation. Whether or not she's still wearing panties, start by simply placing the palm of your hand on her pubic mound. Keep it there for a little while as she begins to wonder what's coming next. If you let your fingers curve right over her mound, she'll feel the warmth of your hand start to stimulate that area. Don't press hard, just cup the mound in your hand. The next move is to stroke her mound softly from top to bottom, in the same way you would stroke a kitten. You can stop for a bit, blow warm air on it, then start stroking again. By this time, she'll be raring for you to rip off her panties. If they're already off, she'll be aching for you to move down lower. If driving her completely wild is on the menu for tonight, you can prolong your teasing by turning your whole hand sideways, and lightly rubbing the edge of it up and down between her legs, over her closed vaginal lips and clit area. Actually, this will feel particularly tantalizing for her if she's still wearing her panties. All these teasing measures are meant to sensitize the entire pubic region, and prime her for what's to come.

The balls of your fingertips are superbly sensitive tools. Dasha prefers fingers over a tongue for the job. "Clitoral stimulation is the best thing," she says. "I really would prefer a man to stroke me with his hands than with his mouth. That's how I usually make myself orgasm. Fingers give me more pleasure than a tongue. The tongue is soft, pliable, whereas fingers are firmer. I like the firmness—it gives me more stimulation." Mercedez echoes this sentiment: "Whether he is giving me oral pleasure or just reaching down, I like fingers."

There are some graphic views of hot hand motion between Dasha's raunchy neighbor and another woman in *One Way Out,* as the camera is set up to catch all the action head-on. After lots of oral action, the two girls position themselves side by side on the sofa. With spread legs and an arm crossed over each other, the camera shoots amazing views of their mutual masturbation. They tweak and rub each other's clit up and down or in a circle. One girl seems to like fingers on her vaginal opening, while the other prefers the focus entirely on her clitoral hood. In this girl-on-girl scene, there are also examples of squeezing the pubic mound and a "fingers-in-clit massage" combo. But one of the actions guys should definitely note is how rapidly they use their hands to brush back and forth over their clits. Their hands shake sideways, very fast, steadily, and with consistent pressure as they bring themselves to orgasm. So, remember to use a slow, light hand in the beginning, and a rapid, steady one toward the end.

Bobby offers men some solid advice on touching. "Rubbing the inside of her thighs, then etching the outline of her pussy with your fingers—and then go back up and kiss her, but use your knee to rub on her clit. You've already rubbed all over her body, so she's all hot and bothered. If you really dig your woman and want to fulfill her, you have to find some fantasies she has. And if you're good at what you do, she'll be ready for you to do whatever next."

G-Spot Stimulation

❝ ❝ **I'm a big fan of stimulation and penetration with someone's hand. Start with one and then two fingers, and then go hard. I love it when someone works my G-spot. ❞ ❞**

—*Mercedez*

Manual penetration is also a perfect way to find a woman's G-spot. The G-spot is another name for the urethral sponge, the spongy tissue around the urethra, the tube that leads from the bladder to the hole we pee through. The G-spot is located about one inch inside the vagina and toward the front of her body, and you can feel the sponge through the vaginal wall. The G-spot swells as a woman gets turned on, so it becomes more prominent and easier to find. G-spot stimulation can vary, but as a general rule, it must be firm and deliberate. Many people like the "come-here" technique, where you insert a finger or two with your palm facing upward, then curve your fingers toward you as if beckoning someone to your side. Continue this motion as you firmly press against the G-spot. Others prefer a pulling motion, where you locate the spot, then move your fingers in and out slightly as if trying to pull it out of her body. Another trick is to use your forefinger and middle finger, and alternate your strokes between the two, as if your fingers are "walking" on her G-spot. For a good look at a guy working his way toward a girl's G-spot, take a look at an early scene in *Student Body* with Dasha and the professor, who shows off his wealth of knowledge.

"A lot of guys will take their fingers and stick them straight in you, but men who know what they are doing curve their fingers to aim toward my G-spot—that feels really good," says Kira. Most women say that they feel like they have to pee when their G-spot is stimulated, which makes sense since the tissue around the urethra is very sensitive, and triggers a reaction in the urethra. For some, an urge to pee or a full-bladder feeling is extremely pleasurable once they are turned on. For others, no matter how aroused they are, G-spot stimulation is more annoying than anything else. So, like everything else, ask her if she likes it, and if she says yes, inquire about some guidance; after all, she knows her body best! If your partner enjoys G-spot stimulation, you can also try curved dildos or vibrators designed especially for reaching that special spot. Vigorous G-spot stimulation leads to female ejaculation in some women (for more on this topic, see Chapter 11).

Other Strokes

There are outside strokes, inside strokes, and combo strokes. The outside strokes include stroking, rubbing/massaging, tapping, pinching and rolling. In the beginning, stroking on her clit or pussy should be done very delicately; just enough to focus her attention there. Light stroking can be done with or without lubrication as long as it's enticing and not irritating. Massaging and rubbing require her to be somewhat wet.

A pleasurable experience can quickly turn into a painful one if she begins to feel raw. For massaging and rubbing, the motions should be
done slowly and gently in the beginning, with increasing pace and pressure as she gets more aroused. Some women like their partner to begin
with lazy circles that, near the end, get as fast as the motion when you
beat an egg. Another technique is to massage her clit in an up-and-
down motion with the balls of several fingers. This position also en-
ables you to insert the end of your thumb into her vagina at the same
time. This combo massage can also be done with one hand rubbing her
clit, and a finger from the other hand inside. Most women favor a rapid
side-to-side or a diagonal clit rubbing to reach orgasm.

Justin uses several fingers to rub a woman the right way: "I like
putting two to three fingers over the mound, just over the clitoral
hood, with the tops of my fingers just at her opening. I rub in a circular motion with just the tips of my fingers." He learned and per-
fected his techniques by going straight to the best source of
information: "If you really want to find out what turns a girl on, have
her masturbate in front of you." If your girl is game, this is a great way
to see exactly how she likes her clitoris stimulated. Have her go slow,
and maybe tell you what she's doing; pay attention to the motion of
her fingers, the amount of pressure she applies, and the position she
likes to be in while she does it. Then you can experiment together.

In the orgy scene in Dasha's feature *Unconscious,* you see one of
the women patting her on the mound while one of the male actors
penetrates her. In Sunrise's film *Filthy Rich,* there is a good clit-
tapping scene between the lawyer and one of the money-hungry
daughters. Gentle rhythmic tapping with an open hand right on the
top of the mound sends little shock waves of stimulation all around
the pubic area. Periodic tapping can also be fun, just as long as it
doesn't turn into slapping. Every subtle movement of your hand is
transmitted in tiny vibrations through her vulva and clitoris. Move
your hand back and forth, gradually increasing the speed of the motion until you are "vibrating" your hand as fast as you can. This light
but focused touch helps the clitoris and entire genital region to

become engorged and swell. It's a great way to get a woman ready, or begging, for more, although many women can orgasm from manual clitoral stimulation alone.

Another motion to tease her clit is light pinching, or pinching and twirling. The pressure with which you can pinch depends on how hard her clit has become. But the basic action of taking her clit between your thumb and forefinger, squeezing it a bit, then rolling it gently between your fingers can be a nice interlude for her. It can also be helpful if your hand is getting tired from lots of rubbing.

For inside moves, venture down from her clitoris and slide a finger between her lips. Lube your fingers with her wetness (add some lube if necessary), and slide some of the lubricant back up over her clit. Part her labia with your finger, going up and down. This will spread her natural lubrication around and also stimulate her clit. It's quite a delicious tease to let that slippery finger slide over the clit slowly, but only for a moment as the finger travels up and down the length of her slit. Vary your speed and the amount of pressure. Find out what she responds to. Briana loves to be teased: "I like when he slides one finger inside, then plays with me, really takes his time before he puts a second finger in. He teases me, goes so slow until I am begging for more."

Some women like the sensation of penetration while you're playing with their clit, and other women prefer to focus all the preliminaries outside and on top, waiting for the penetration of intercourse. Insert just the tip of one finger into her. Feel her vaginal muscles around your finger as you rub her clit with your palm. Move the tip in and out, never going very deep, then move it in a circle, like you're drawing a circle just inside her opening. The opening and just inside the opening are the most sensitive and responsive parts of a woman's vagina. Aim your index finger like you're pointing at something. Guess what you're pointing at? Slide that finger right in there where it is wettest and hottest. You can let your thumb ride up to try to reach her clit as you piston your arm back and forth. You can also make circles with your finger as you pump. For a good view of this "poke-and-stroke" motion, take a look at the scene where the returning girlfriend finds her guy with another woman in *Intimate Journey*. Some women also really love the drilling, twisting motion if you use your thumb, which does not go as deep, but is thicker than your other fingers. This drilling motion, sometimes called "finger fucking" can be a real turn-on, or it can be a real turnoff. Again, try a few different techniques to see what your partner likes best.

Dasha likes the process of relaxing and taking more time. "Start rubbing my clit first, then go inside and continue moving the fingers on my clit from side to side," she says. "Slide two fingers inside, then maybe, after a while, three. Each time you add a finger, I can feel myself relax and open up, taking more and getting more turned on." Justin takes his cues from his partner about when she wants more: "Sometimes she's going to want it gentle; sometimes she's going to want it rough; it all depends. You have to read her body language. I like to just use the tips of my fingers until she starts bucking. That's usually a hint you can go harder."

Here is a technique that feels great, but since the action is mostly happening inside, you won't see it in a film. Start with one finger in her, then switch to your middle finger to get her pussy good and wet. Put both fingers in together and pump them a few times, and add your thumb. Keep the tips of your fingers tightly together for several pumps, but then start opening them as you pull out, and tighten them up again as you go in. Rub her clit with your other hand. Most women agree that you should build up to faster speeds. "I like slow penetration with fingers at first, speed up once I am turned on," says Tawny.

Don't overlook the possibility of combining or alternating between clit stimulation, vaginal penetration, and anal penetration. For any penetration, she must be wet enough to make your finger, or a toy, slide in and out easily. Unlike her vagina, her rectum is not self-lubricating. In Vivid movies, you'll see actors putting their fingers in their own mouths to wet them, spitting some saliva into their hand and applying it, or spitting saliva directly on the anus and rubbing it around a bit. Even when using smooth toys, it's a good idea to use a personal lubricant either on the toy itself or on the body. Check out

Looking In for a slow look at some girl on girl excitement, combining lots of strokes and massages as well as vaginal and anal penetration.

Secrets of Getting and Staying Wet

Some women get wet at the sight of a proud erection, while others will respond merely to a lover's voice. Some need oral sex or other kinds of clitoral stimulation to really get the juices flowing. With many women, the greater the anticipation, the more teasing, the more they self-lubricate. Savanna is one of those women: "It's a sexy idea to be naturally wet. What's really exciting is the anticipation of having sex, of preparing yourself. If you're going on a date, I use my mind all day, thinking about what's going to happen when I finally get the cock. Keeping in that mode, thinking every now and then about what's going to happen, that keeps me wet. Sometimes, by the time it happens I'm almost too wet! It's amazing the effect your mind can have on your pussy." Savanna is right. Our brains are the most important sex organ we've got, and you can start to make yourself wet by thinking about what you expect to happen, imagining what him touching you or sliding into you will be like.

Sometimes, a woman is just wetter or drier than other times. She can be extremely turned on, but not necessarily wet enough to make penetration comfortable. "Sometimes, if I don't have the right foreplay in the beginning, I have trouble getting wet," says Mercedez. "But if it's done like a movie, with lots of going down on each other, then I have no problems. But if I'm not in the mood, and it's kind of rushed, then I definitely have a problem." It's a fact that some women produce more lubrication than others. Sometimes she might feel aroused, but she just doesn't seem to get very wet. A guy might think he's doing a poor job, or that she's not interested, but there are a variety of factors that can affect a woman's ability to naturally lubricate, including: dehydration, drinking alcohol or smoking marijuana, her menstrual cycle, stress, illness, or getting older. A lack of lubrication can also be a side effect of many common prescription and over-the-counter medications, including some birth control pills, antihistamines, and cold or allergy medicines. Kira has this dilemma: "It's tough for me to stay wet, because my pills dry me out. So you have to know how to switch gears. One night we can be going rough, but then switching gears to kissing me lightly can really get me going. Keeping up the foreplay and using lube are what work for me." You might want to take a look at *The Kiss*. There are several long scenes in this film, including three different boy-girl combinations and one all-girl threesome, that are good examples of lubing things up while keeping the scene sexy.

Personal Lubricants

❝ ❝ Before I started performing in movies, I didn't use lube, but now, not only do I use it all the time, I don't like the feeling of sex without it. A really good lube makes sex more comfortable and keeps you going. ❞ ❞

—Mercedez

Some women will start out with lots of natural fluid, but as penetration progresses, their bodies don't produce enough fluid to keep up with the action. Plus, lube is a necessity for anal penetration. (Read more about anal pleasure in Chapter 10.) The most important thing to remember is that if she's not wet enough, it doesn't necessarily mean she doesn't want to have sex or that she's not turned on. The solution is easy: use a personal lubricant.

Personal lubricants are an irreplaceable staple on the set of Vivid movies, and they should be on your bedside table as well! Think about it: most sexual activities are about rubbing parts of your body against parts of your partner's body or penetration, all of which produce friction. Lubricants make everything slide in and out more easily and thus make all kinds of sex better. Penetration without proper lubrication is not only uncomfortable, it can actually hurt. "Sometimes, after a few minutes of having intercourse . . . you're dehydrated," notes

Dasha. "Always keep the lube around. You can really hurt yourself if you have sex when you are dry."

On occasion, if foreplay is rushed, lube can help ease the transition to intercourse: "Sometimes if I don't have enough foreplay in the beginning, I have trouble getting wet," says Briana. "That's why lube is great." For some women, initial lubrication is fine, but the longer intercourse lasts, the more they need a "boost" to keep going.

If you are playing with vibrators or other sex toys, which are made of rubber, silicone, or other materials, lube will make them feel better against your skin or inside you. Likewise, if you are practicing safer sex, using a latex barrier, gloves, and/or condoms, Savanna reminds you that lube is essential: "Especially when you use condoms, you absolutely need lube. The latex dries up your natural lubrication." The same is true for nonlatex products as well, so lubricant should be considered part of your safer sex arsenal.

Remember, too, that lube is not just for intercourse; it adds something to hand jobs for both him and her, making skin-on-skin contact slick, slippery, and extremely pleasurable. But some women caution you about using too much lube. "If I use too much lube, then I can't feel the penetration as well, there isn't enough friction," says Mercedez. "Don't overdo it. You have to put just a few drops. If there's too much then it's annoying, and it doesn't feel good, either."

A Guide to Lube

❝❝ I used to be ashamed, because I thought he's going to think he's not turning me on or he's not sexy to me if I am not wet. You just have to tell your guy, 'You turn me on so much, but I guess my body is dehydrated and so I need some lube.' Girls shouldn't be ashamed of using lube. ❞❞

—Dasha

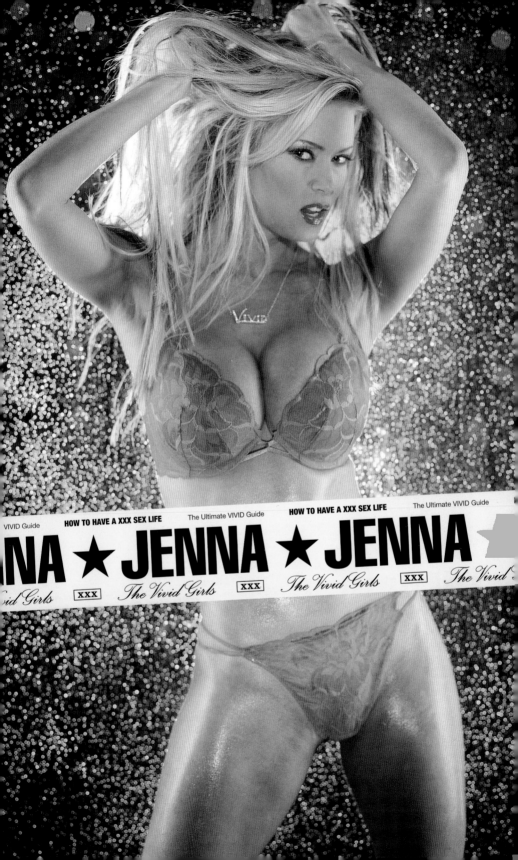

NA ★ JENNA ★ JENNA ★

id Girls   XXX   The Vivid Girls   XXX   The Vivid Girls   XXX   The Vivid

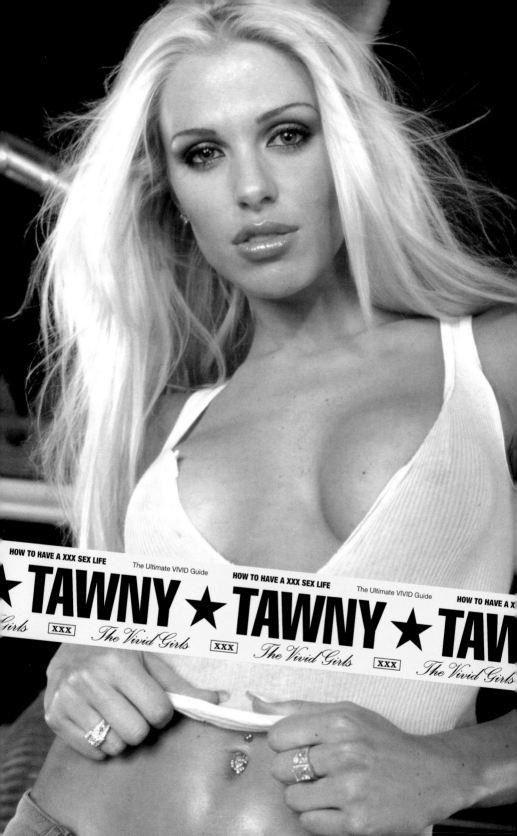

HOW TO HAVE A XXX SEX LIFE The Ultimate VIVID Guide HOW TO HAVE A XXX SEX LIFE The Ultimate VIVID Guide HOW TO HAVE A X

TAWNY ★ **TAWNY** ★ **TAW**

Girls XXX *The Vivid Girls* XXX *The Vivid Girls* XXX *The Vivid Girls*

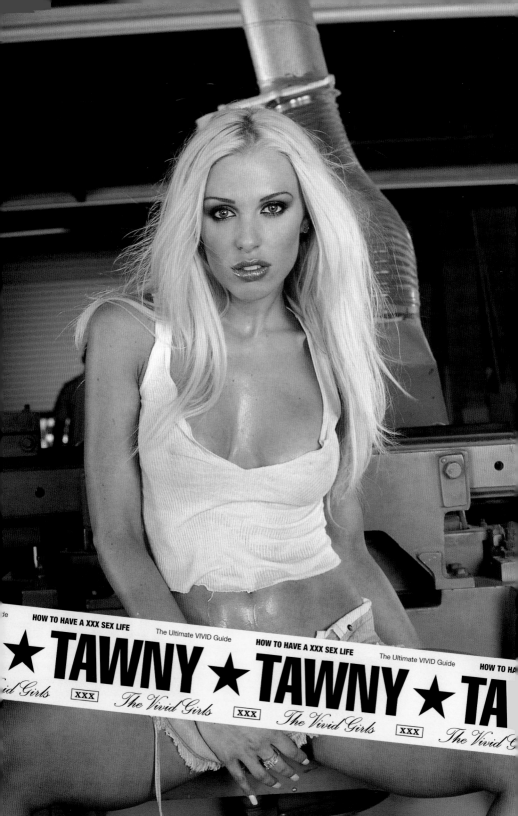

★ **TAWNY** ★ **TAWNY** ★ **TA**

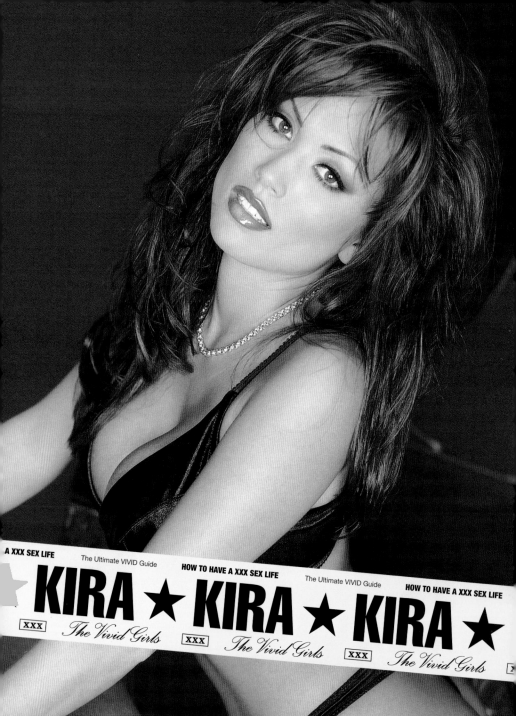

A XXX SEX LIFE   The Ultimate VIVID Guide   HOW TO HAVE A XXX SEX LIFE   The Ultimate VIVID Guide   HOW TO HAVE A XXX SEX LIFE

KIRA ★ KIRA ★ KIRA ★

XXX *The Vivid Girls*   XXX *The Vivid Girls*   XXX *The Vivid Girls*

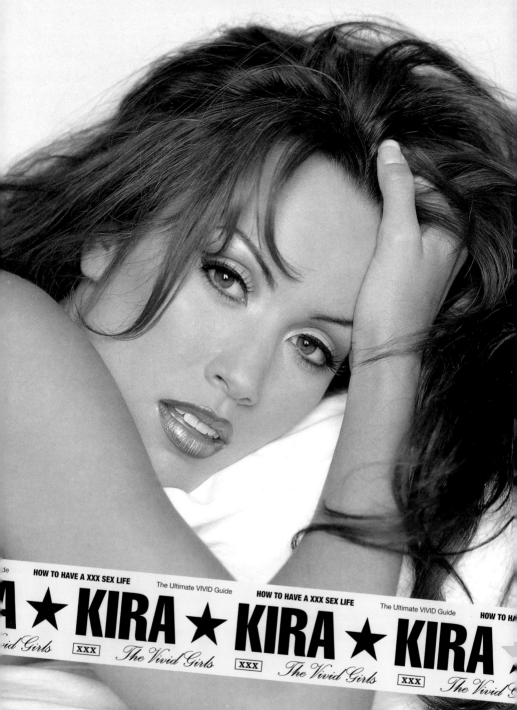

 ★ KIRA ★ KIRA ★ KIRA

HOW TO HAVE A XXX SEX LIFE   The Ultimate VIVID Guide   HOW TO HAVE A XXX SEX LIFE   The Ultimate VIVID Guide   HOW TO HA

The Vivid Girls   XXX   *The Vivid Girls*   XXX   *The Vivid G*

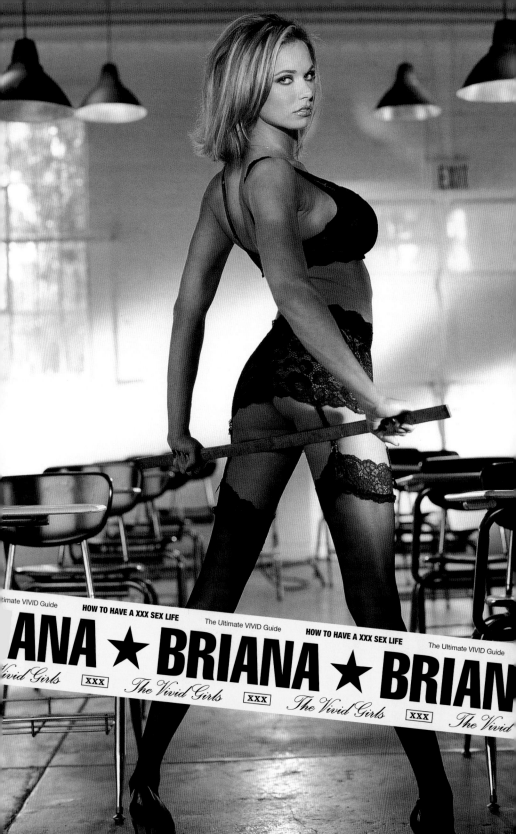

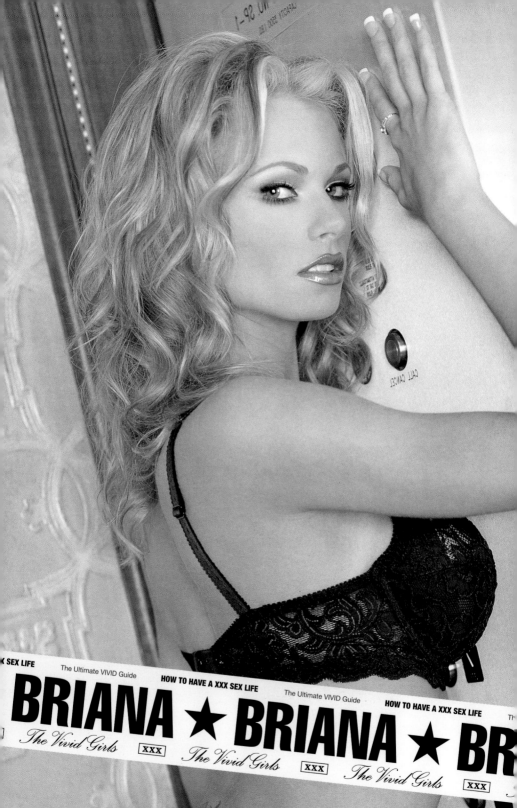

DASHA ★ DASHA ★ DASH

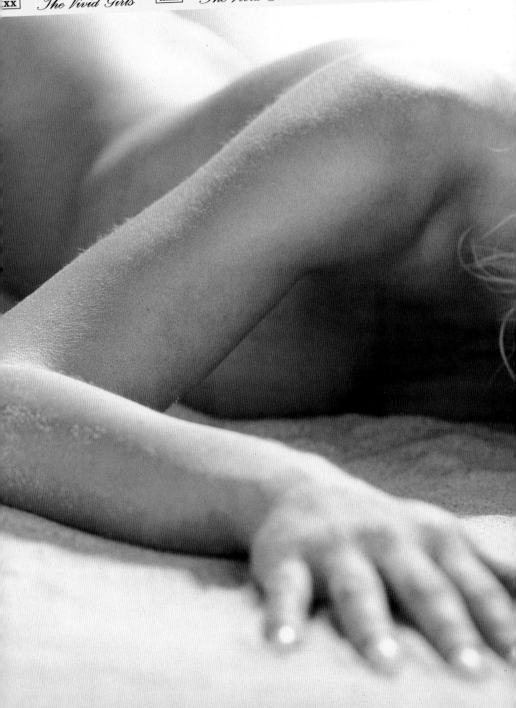

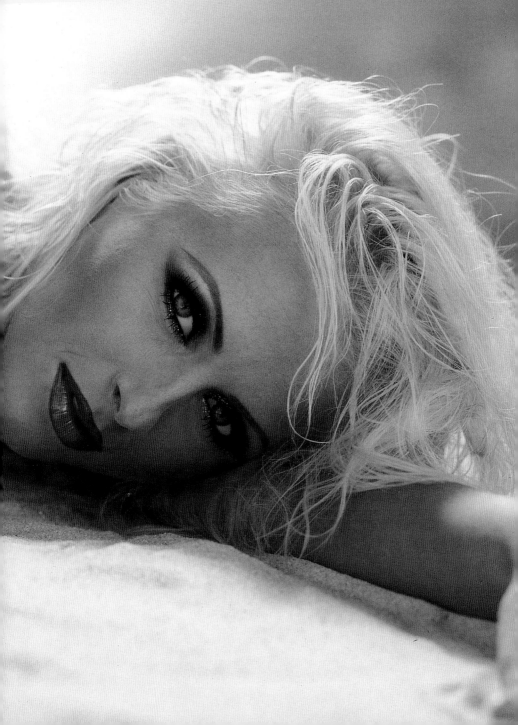

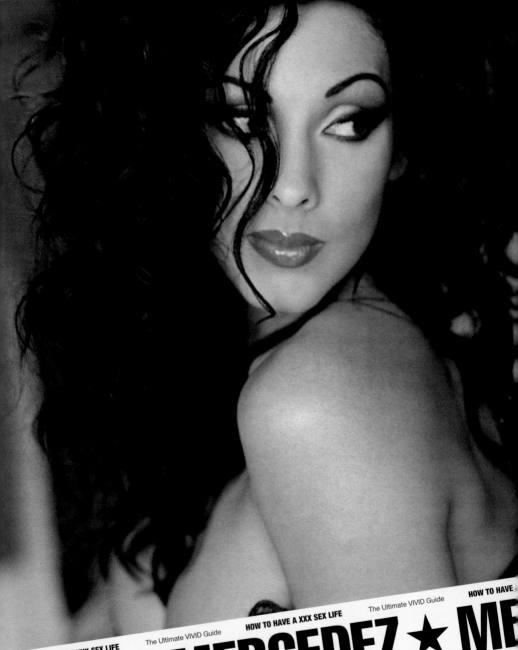

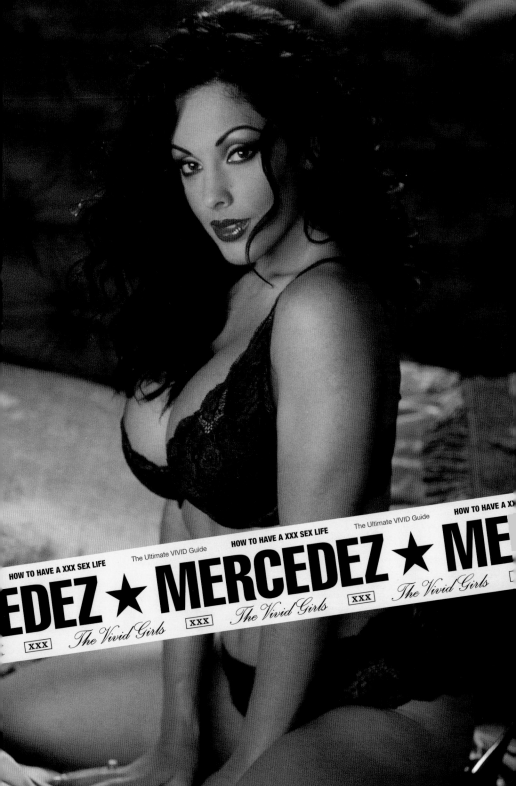

EDEZ ★ MERCEDEZ ★ ME

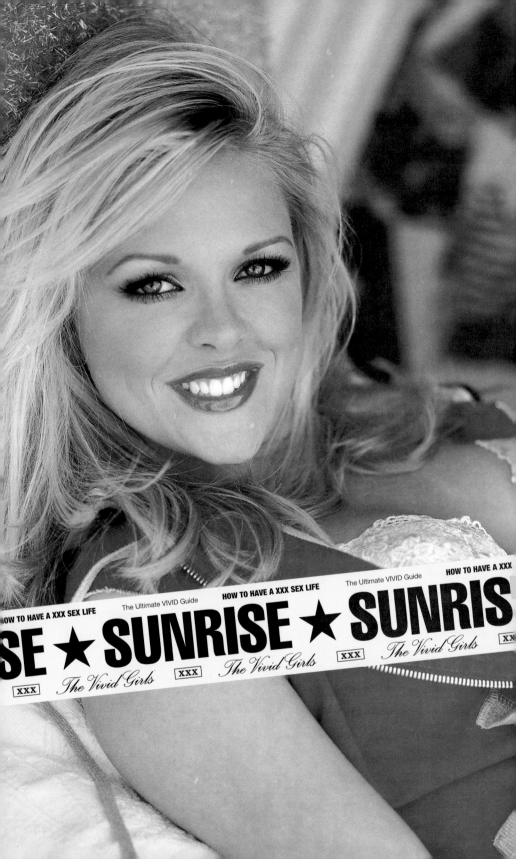

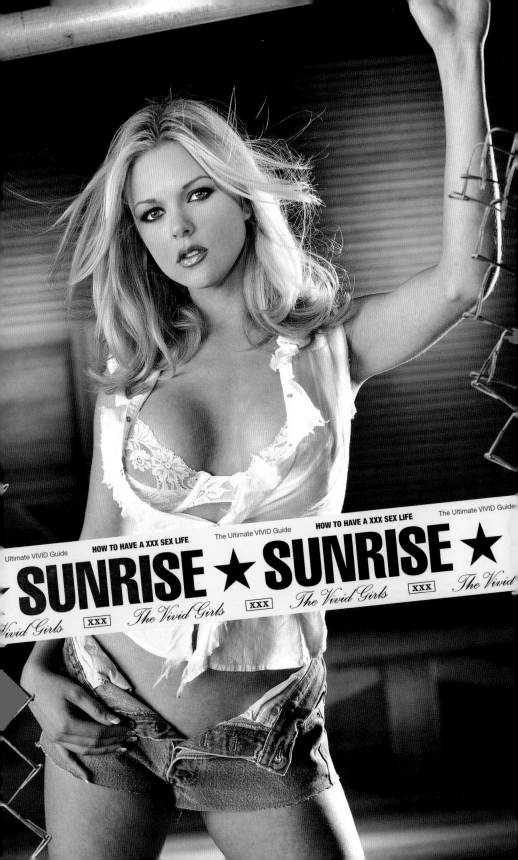

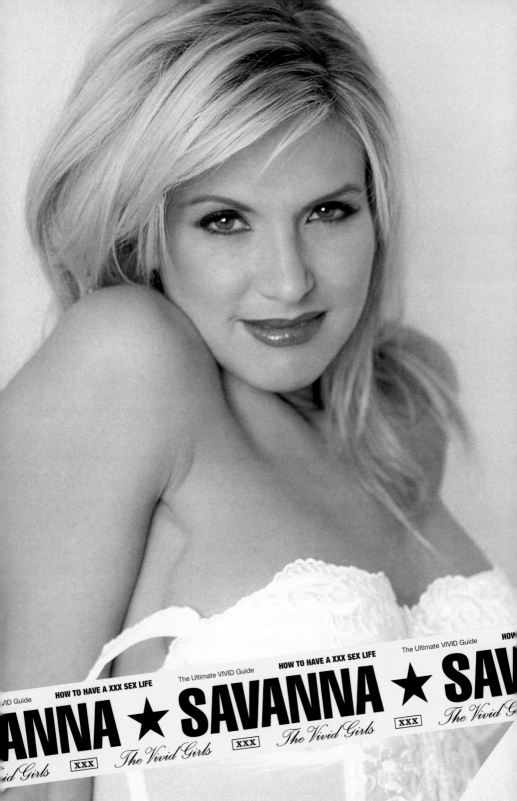

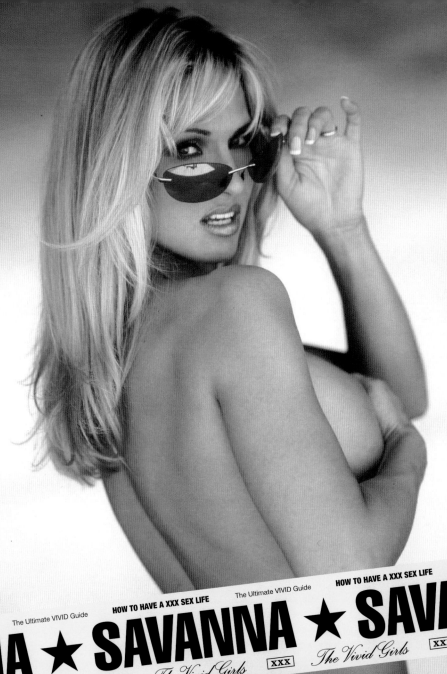

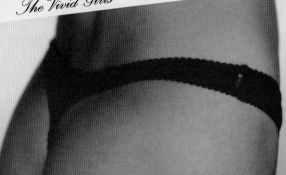

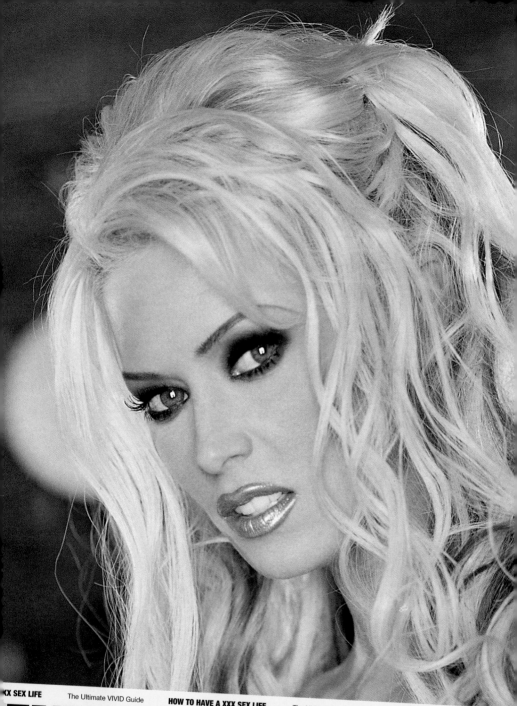

ENNA ★ JENNA ★ JENNA

You don't want to substitute household products for lube, so things like vegetable or olive oil, lotions and moisturizers, hair conditioners, cosmetic creams, Vaseline, baby oil—all of which most men have probably used to toss off at one time or another—can be harsh on the vaginal tissue, cause an allergic reaction, or give women a bad yeast, bacterial, or other infection. The same goes for food items like whipped cream, butter, honey, or chocolate sauce; they are fine for spreading on external parts, but never put them inside any orifices!

There are so many different kinds of lubricants on the market that everyone should be able to find one that's perfect for them. Personal lubricants are so popular today that you'll probably find at least one or two brands at the pharmacy, either near the condoms, or in the aisle near the "feminine" products. If you can't obtain personal lubricants easily, try the Internet. But to determine just which product is right for you, we suggest you visit your local sex-toy store, buy several sample packets, and try them all out. We can't think of a better research assignment than that.

Water-based lubes are latex-safe, easy to clean up, and come in a variety of consistencies from slick (meant to mimic natural vaginal lubrication) to thick (better for anal sex). Most water-based lubricants contain glycerin, the ingredient that helps them "stay wet." When the lube dries up, you can add a little water or spit to revive it. Some water-based brands include AstroGlide, Elbow Grease, ForPlay, ID Glide, K-Y, Probe, Sex Grease, and Wet. "I definitely have a variety of lubes on the set, as well as nonlatex condoms, because someone can be allergic," says Chi Chi. "I'm not a big person for flavored lubes. I don't want to taste cinnamon, I want to taste human."

If you or your partner gets easily irritated, or has frequent yeast infections, then you may be sensitive or allergic to glycerin. There are water-based lubes that have most of the same properties and ingredients as others minus the glycerin. Look for names like Hydra Smooth, Liquid Silk, Maximus, Sensual Power, and Slippery Stuff. These lubes tend to dry up more quickly, so you'll need to relube more often.

Silicone-based lubes, like Eros, I-D Millennium, Wet Platinum, and Domestic Partners' DP Glide, are compatible with latex and are not absorbed into the body, so they don't dry up like water-based lubes. Most silicone lubes are thin and slippery, allowing for plenty of friction. You also need a much smaller amount to get the job done since they are super-long-lasting. One caution: silicone lube ruins CyberSkin and silicone sex toys, so they should never be used together.

Last, we remind you that everyone has his or her preferences regarding fragrance. Finding a lube that's perfectly scented for both of you shouldn't be too hard. But if you can't agree, we suggest fragrance-free lube. Whether your girl is always slippery when wet or she needs a boost, lube is one ingredient you can add to make your sex life better.

When tall, blond, and gorgeous Dasha landed in America, she had the same ambition that many immigrants do: to make a better life for herself. Since she had just a tentative grasp of English, the only job she could get was as a janitor at a Kmart in Washington, D.C. The baggy overalls she wore concealed her extraordinary beauty and she had few prospects. She was soon promoted to the position of manager, but thought there must be something better. Desperate to improve her life, she and a friend bought a beat up car and drove to Hollywood, where she became a dancer in a topless bar. Still living in her car on the beach in Santa Monica, she decided she needed a more lucrative job. She visited an adult video store and began looking at the box covers of the features on display. Vivid Video, she discovered, had the most attractive covers. She jotted down the street address of the Vivid office in Van Nuys and drove there the next day, presenting herself at the office and asking for a job application. The receptionist took one look at Dasha and called one of her bosses to come out and meet her. The rest is history. After Dasha was signed as a Vivid Girl, her first movie, *Broken English,* was a bestseller. As one of the top adult film stars, Dasha has found success and happiness plus love and romance. She met her current husband, actor Dillon Day, on the set of a movie.

Working in adult movies has been very fulfilling for Dasha, who says she enjoys the chance to expand her own erotic horizons as well those of the people who watch her movies at home. "There are so many things I never tried before I did them in films, and I definitely have had great experiences, like sex with another woman, and a ménage à trois. Working in the adult industry has given me a broader view of sexuality." Although she said she likes being with women, she much prefers men. When Dasha was asked who, besides her husband, she most looked forward to working with, she replied Bobby Vitale. "Being a Vivid Girl has allowed me to do what I like to do, have amazing sex, be in front of the camera, and do it with style. Vivid is tops; who wouldn't enjoy it?"

Dasha recommends films to anyone who wants to try something new. "Movies are great to get you excited, but they can also give you ideas and inspiration to do things you hadn't even considered before. All the things we do in the movies are not that difficult. It's pretty easy for people to figure out how to do it; just study the positions. I was raised by strict parents, and didn't know a lot about sex. I had no idea where my clitoris was until I saw a woman touching herself in a movie! When I discovered clitoral stimulation, that changed everything!"

Dasha says her most memorable movie is *Highway 1*. "I liked the story and I had great sex," she says. Surprisingly, Dasha's favorite moments in a scene don't come at the climax. "I like teasing the guy before he's totally aroused, looking into his eyes, seeing him get excited. Teasing before you let him touch you is the best part. The eyes are the sexiest part of a man. I love it when a guy can look at you and say everything with his eyes: 'You're beautiful and amazing and I want you so bad!' I'm there."

"That's how my husband got me," she says. "I was filming my second movie, and Dillon was my costar. We were in missionary position, and he just kept staring into my eyes. He was communicating so much through his eyes, a passion and depth that amazed me. After that scene, we started dating." Dasha says, "I admire sensitive, ambitious, respectable men . . . Dillon is that way."

In her home life, Dasha strives to keep things fresh and

interesting. "I'm one of those people who likes a routine: we eat dinner, we watch television, we get ready for bed, then we have sex. But my husband doesn't always want sex to be on a schedule. So sometimes when we are getting ready to go somewhere, even if we are in a hurry, I'll just rip his pants off and pounce on him! Or when he's on the phone, I'll drop to my knees and surprise him. I want to pat myself on the back when I do. It's fun to do anything that's unexpected or out of the usual pattern. Sometimes, it's work, but spontaneity keeps you on your toes."

In addition to her work in the adult entertainment industry, Dasha caught the attention of mainstream producers and was cast in the Deftones' long-form video *Change*, and then in the album artwork and music video for Warner Brothers recording artist Brougham. In addition, Madonna picked her for a spot in her "Music" video. Dasha has modeled for the famous photographer David LaChapelle, and has been featured in such fashion books as *Flaunt* and *Dune* (Japan). She was also selected by *Playboy* for a pictorial on top adult stars.

Widely appreciated for her classic European beauty and elegance, Dasha draws packed audiences when she appears as a featured dancer at gentlemen's clubs around the country. *Exotic Dancer* magazine, the trade bible of the gentlemen's club circuit, selected her as its Adult Movie Feature Entertainer of the Year (2002).

When not performing, Dasha enjoys ballroom dancing, horseback riding, swimming, lots of exercise, and cooking. She loves watching the Discovery Channel; her favorite TV shows have been *The Simpsons*, *Married with Children*, *M.A.S.H.*, and *I Love Lucy*, and her favorite colors are pink and purple. And what's her favorite music? "I like all kinds of music," she says. "Enya, Whitney Houston, Andrea Bocelli, Metallica, and even country music."

VIVID FEATURES STARRING DASHA (RELEASED AS OF 11-25-03)

- Broken English
- Student Body
- Highway 1
- Highway 2
- The Big Bust
- Shakespeare Revealed
- Dreams
- Snapshot
- Now or Never
- Unconscious
- Morning Star
- Angel
- Where the Boys Aren't 14
- Where the Boys Aren't 15
- Upper Class
- Take 5
- Wifetaker
- Hot Orchid
- Shy
- Heaven's Revenge
- Dashed
- Liquid Sex
- Perfection
- Photo Club
- The Alley
- One Way Out
- Nailed

DASHA STATS:

Birthplace: Czech Republic
Birth date: November 21
Heritage: Czech
Sign: Scorpio
Measurements: 34C–25–34
Eyes: Hazel green
Hair: Blond
Height: 5'9''
Weight: 130

8
knock on wood

Fantasy File:

Not one hour ago, Jerry and his best buddy Frank were sitting alone bored in his house. Now, with some help from a world-famous illusionist, the two men are sitting in a room with some of the sexiest women from history, and their three dream women of all time: Cleopatra, Helen of Troy, and Delilah. Cleopatra is a vision in gold and black, a voluptuous beauty with intense kohl-rimmed eyes and jet-black hair topped by a gold headdress with a large ruby in the center. Helen of Troy is blond and sensuous, her hair piled loosely on her head, with a necklace of many chains highlighting the graceful curve of her neck. Tall and slender in her red platform heels, Delilah is mouthy, forceful, and controlling. Soon she demands to see their "swords" and Cleopatra pulls Jerry's penis out of his pants. Not overly impressed with his manhood, Cleopatra takes him in her mouth to see how big he can get. Everyone else in the room watches as she kneels before him and slowly sucks his cock.

Impatient for more, Delilah snaps, "Cleo, you may have ruled Egypt, but you couldn't fuck your way out of a paper sack. Let me show you how it's done." She grabs Jerry, his pants gathered around his ankles, and throws him back on the sofa. Unaccustomed to being tossed around by a girl, Jerry isn't sure he likes it. At the same time, though, he feels himself becoming more and more aroused as she takes more and more control. Leaning back on the sofa, Jerry opens his legs for more attention. Delilah snaps up her long flowing skirt, squats down before him, and takes hold of his penis with a startlingly strong hand.

As Jerry watches in wide-eyed amazement, she takes nearly of all his now huge cock into her mouth. She massages his dick roughly with her hand, then goes back down on him. He's never seen a woman suck cock like this. She spits on his dick with a loud smacking noise to lube him up for her handiwork. With her mouth on the head of his penis, she pivots her hand back and forth as she moves up and down the shaft. She spits on him again, then takes his rock-hard rod in both hands. She clasps her hands together and interlocks her fingers, pushing his penis through the slippery tunnel formed by her hands. It feels better than any hand job he's ever had before, more forceful and more exciting at the same time.

His cock is one big pole of sensation as he feels her hands move across every millimeter of the shaft and head. She pushes his cock all the way to the back of her throat; he feels a little glimmer of pride that she still can't take in the whole length at once. She pulls away, then glides her slippery lips down to his balls, then flicks them from side to side with her tongue.

Delilah pulls back as she removes her dress, unleashing her large, perfectly round breasts of biblical-epic proportions. She massages her nipples with the tips of her fingers, then leans forward onto Jerry. She presses her breasts together around his cock. His dick stands straight up as she envelops him in her soft pillows. Still wrapped around him, she begins to bob her whole body up and down so that his cock is fucking her tits. He lets out a long slow exhale. Given the pleasures of history's sexiest siren, all he can manage to say is "aahh, fuck yeah." She could make him shoot his load in an instant, but she wants more. She leaves Jerry and moves on to Frank. On her hands and knees in front of him,

she points her perky bottom up in the air, wordlessly inviting
Jerry to explore the historic pleasures of her pussy . . .

★★ *from* The Vision,
directed by Cleo Edwards

In the lusty world of adult entertainment, a hand job may seem like small potatoes compared to hot group scenes, acrobatic intercourse, and anal sex. But let's not forget that just about all sex, whether in real life or captured on film, begins with manual action. A sex-starved vixen may hungrily pull the penis out of a guy's pants, or a college coed can tentatively massage her man's groin, but the bottom line is the same. "Real" sex begins when the girl grabs the guy's dick. So before diving in, a few Vivid pointers for women on handling the male member.

Getting to know the male member is an important part of becoming a top-notch lover. For women, discovering your guy's special preferences and what turns him on most is a significant step in building the bond between the two of you. Since most women haven't a clue about erections, we'll start with them.

Getting Wood

❝ ❝ Give him a lot of attention. Be very giving, mentally and physically. I appreciate a lot of energy and focus. ❞ ❞

—Paul Thomas

Just as sustained intercourse requires the woman to be wet, it requires the guy to be hard. And, just as a woman's wetness is not necessarily an indicator of how aroused she is, so a man's hard-on is not necessarily an indicator of his degree of arousal. Some guys get hard and can stay that way for what seems like hours. Others need constant attention, or very specific attention, to maintain their "wood"—that's porno slang for "erection."

Bobby talks seriously about getting erections on cue for the camera. "A lot of buff guys come into the business and say, 'Yeah, my dick gets hard when the wind blows.' But when they are doing their twentieth scene with the same girl, can they get it up? The girl could be the prettiest thing in the world but a complete bitch, and how do you get it up then? Some people you're going to have chemistry with and some you're not. Some don't do it for me, and with girls, not every guy does it for them."

As anyone who's ever read a Viagra label knows, arousal is an important part of an erection. Nothing can get a guy hard if he simply isn't into it. Kira notes that feeling desired is always an important part of being aroused, so what you *say* to a man can be as significant as what you *do* to him. She adds, "Cater to his ego. Talk about how big or beautiful his cock is, how much you love it and want it, how much he turns you on." On the preliminaries, Mercedez agrees that a little verbal addition can help get a guy going. "Sometimes I talk to him and tell him dirty stories or how bad I want it. I tell him what I'm going to do once he gets hard. I'll tell him what kind of blow job I'm going to give and then I'll do it once he gets it up."

To make your erection connection a success, Team Vivid again emphasizes the power of the tease. "It's important that a girl keeps eye contact. Always know how your body looks sexy. If you see him going a little soft, maybe go down on him, kiss up and down his neck, whisper to him. Most guys, once it's up, it's up—just keep the mood going and tease, tease, tease," says Justin. Sometimes you can get wood without even touching the penis. Instead, focus on the areas all around it: move your hands up and down his thighs, brush your lips near his dick without touching it. His anticipation of what's to come should cause his mini-me to jump right up. While you're teasing him, take his hand in yours and place it on his dick, then watch how he handles himself for a few minutes. Jenna is another devotee of watch and learn. "I like watching guys masturbate. I watch exactly how they do it, and then I know what they like, and how to do it to them," she says.

If you encounter erection problems, go for the tried-and-true.

How did you get him hard the first time? Did you stroke him a little? Lick him? If he wasn't already bursting out of his pants, then think back to what you did then and it will probably work again. The important thing to remember is that even the pros can lose a hard-on. If a deflation (or lack of inflation) comes your way, Sunrise suggests patience and understanding. "I love to get to inside people's heads and find out what makes them tick. If you can't really read them, they are going to go limp. Before you start, you have to get to know his body and then play with that. If you start looking away and acting bored, he'll lose it. Stay in tune with him, stare into his eyes. Show him that you are there for him, that it's a two-person thing maintaining an erection. A lot of guys get embarrassed and feel really bad about themselves. You just have to say that you're there, you're willing to help them out, and that it's okay to have problems."

Rings and Things

Cock rings are another tool to help keep a guy hard. Many women find them totally sexy these days, especially with their bad-boy connotations. And it's a great little gift for Valentine's Day. Rings are made in many materials, including steel, rubber, leather, and that rubber jelly material often used in sex toys. The way they work is by keeping all the extra blood that rushes into a guy's member for a hard-on where you want it: in his dick. The kind with snaps is often preferred because the guy can quickly unsnap it when he's ready to let loose his load, and you don't have to wait to take it off after coming, as is often the case with solid steel or rubber rings. As an added bonus, for many guys, cock rings keep them so rock hard that it intensifies feeling all up and down the dick.

Hand Jobs for Him

The pleasures of a good hand job should not be overlooked. You can begin before you even get into his pants. Run your whole hand over his crotch and chances are you'll feel some wood underneath already, especially if you've already been kissing. Jenna recommends a gentle touch at first. "In my experience, I think it's sexier for a guy when a girl is kind of gentle about playing with his dick. I know if I had a penis, I wouldn't want some girl grabbing it and yanking on it," she adds. Another hot Jenna "woodymaker" tip: "A good way to start is when you go down and he still has his shorts on, and you breathe so he can feel your breath through the shorts." In *Filthy Rich,* scheming daughter Jessica Nelson makes a play for the probate lawyer and does exactly that. She kneels on the sofa in front of him and massages his groin through his pants. Then she breathes on the area and even licks him lightly. In your scenes, once the pants come off, and they will very soon, you can continue to tease him just a bit by massaging around his thighs and pelvis. Dasha says, "I like to play around the pubic area, the base of his penis, and start sliding up and down. Make sure your hand is wet or lubed up enough so you don't hurt him."

As things heat up, you can deliver a light dry stroke in the classic ring formation made by wrapping your thumb and index finger around his shaft. Use a light touch, which can be very tantalizing, in the same way that a very light back-scratching with your fingernails feels. But once you're ready to really stroke, you'll need some lubrication. "Don't stroke a guy dry," says Justin. "Use lube, or if you have good spit, use that." Rubbing hard while a guy is still dry can cause unpleasant friction. For hand work, use a thin, slick lube, since the thicker brands can get too gooey. It's also a good idea to select one that doesn't get sticky right away, because that will interfere with your smooth sliding ability. Tawny likes to make the lubing up part of the whole sexperience. "Use your mouth to spit on it," she recommends. "Even if you're also using lubricant. It not only lubes him up, but it can be really sexy to lick him, lick your hand, all the while looking at him."

To hand-tailor your hand job, Justin recommends watching the guy do it to himself. "Have the guy masturbate in front of you and watch how he moves his hand. Mimic what he does and don't be afraid to ask: How does this feel? Do you like that? Ask him what he likes and doesn't like." The stroke styles are seemingly endless. We've seen guys use a two-hand grip, a full hand around the full shaft, those who handle just the tip, and those who make a ring like we described earlier.

Once you're both properly lubricated, slide your hand up and down, from the base of his penis all the way up the ridge where the head flares out. The most sensitive part of the shaft is that spot just under the ridge. "I put my thumb on the V of the head, that's the most sensitive part, and use my thumb to stimulate it as I move my hand up and down," says Savanna.

Another style is to use your whole hand in a pumping motion, but instead of stopping at the head, keep going all way up and over it. As with most of your techniques, start slowly and then increase the speed. Briana is a fan of the "tunnel-of-love" hand job. "I interlace my fingers and thumbs and make a hole in my hands to jerk him off that way," she says. But, she warns, "Don't wear your rings if you do that maneuver. They just don't feel good for the guy." On uncircumcised guys, you can use the extra foreskin near the head to add a little extra tug while stroking. The looser skin of on uncircumcised guy can also be held loosely in your hand while you let the harder shaft underneath glide through it almost like a sleeve. Most American men are circumcised, while most European men aren't, but it's a good technique to have up your sleeve should you find yourself caught up in international relations.

As always, pay close attention to his reactions. "Sometimes you can just feel a guy jump and you've done something he doesn't like, even if he won't say so out loud," says Briana. On the flip side, adds Tawny, "I can usually tell by the expression on his face if likes what I'm doing. If he looks like he's in ecstasy, then I keep doing what I'm doing." If he really enjoys manual stimulation, the girls recommend lubing up both hands and making a Briana-style tunnel. You can pump your interlaced hands up and down on him, or hold steady and let him thrust through them. Other bonus moves: squeezing very tight; varying the pressure by squeezing harder or softer at different points along the penis; and rotating your hands in opposite directions as you move up and down. *Filthy Rich's* Jessica, mentioned above, does a two-hand twist with opposite rotation on the probate lawyer's shaft while sucking on the head. Of course it helps that his superhard cock is long and fat enough to accommodate not only both her hands but her mouth, too.

Yet another exciting sensation comes from using your nails. Justin says, "I like the look of fingernails, and I like the feel of them on my body lightly. When you use them, tease with them, rake them down my body." Your fingernails will feel totally different than your fingertips, and many men find them very sexy (another reason for all those perfect manicures on the Vivid Girls). You can brush your nails lightly along his penis, but feel free to use them anywhere else you can reach with one hand while stroking his dick with the other.

Handball

Just as we said not to neglect the balls during oral sex, you shouldn't forget them during a hand job either. Justin says women should always pay attention to a guy's balls. Just remember, that the balls are extremely sensitive, so play gently, at least at first. Ball play works well even during intercourse. In the retro-futuristic drama *Domination Nation,* men go into hiding because they die after they ejaculate. In the last scene, the good woman scientist finally gets to have sex with a real man. While sitting on his dick, she reaches back and gently massages his balls as he thrusts up into her. For straight-on manual action, use your fingers and the palm of your hand to cup the balls and lift them up while you are stroking his shaft with the other hand. You can even squeeze them lightly. Let's repeat that just to make sure you got it: *lightly.* Some guys like it a bit rougher, but all the Vivid Girls advise asking before you go there. "I had one boyfriend who really loved being scratched under his balls, but since then all the other guys are scared," says Dasha. Using your fingertips or fingernails, gently scratch upward from underneath the balls, all way back near his ass, then continue up toward the penis. If he likes the feel of this, the loose skin around the balls may tighten up, which is a sign that he may be close to coming. The cock ring can come in handy during ball play, too. With a cock ring, the skin around the ball sac is usually tighter, so the whole package becomes easier to handle and less fragile than when the balls are dangling loosely.

Talented multitaskers all, the Vivid Girls are big fans of using your hands and mouth at the same time on the balls. In *Student Body*, talented Tri Twat girl Julie gives her tutor a special send off before he heads to Oxford on an international exchange program. Seated side by side on a bench on the leafy green campus, she leans over and does some awesome extra-credit work. While sucking his cock, she cups her hand underneath his balls, then brings them up into position for sucking. First one ball and then the other, followed by a long lick from the base of his balls all the way up to the top of his penis. Once you've got your oral and manual skills down, the combination of the two should blow his mind.

★ **BONUS** ★
★ **POINTS:**

WARM WET WASHCLOTH

While we all seem to enjoy the big money shot in a porn film, what should a girl do tidy up afterward? The covered-in-cum look may be hot image on film, but it can be messy, especially if it dries on you overnight. While this subject is definitely not covered in Emily Post, the best etiquette for postcoital cum cleanup is to discreetly mop it up. Take a hand towel or washcloth and run part of it under hot water from the sink. Kindly Nurse Tang does it for the sex fiend patient in her care after they finally get it on in *Nurses*. Use the moist part to wipe off your face, chest, or other covered parts, then gently rub any excess off *his* belly, thighs, or wherever else it may have ended up. It's a nice gesture, and the warm towel feels pretty good, too, especially after a vigorous lovemaking session.

Up Close & Personal
★ Savanna Samson ★

Blond bombshell Savanna Samson grew up in a small town in upstate New York where she was one of five sisters. She belies every stereotype of the porn star except two—she's gorgeous and very sexy. As with most Libras, Savanna loves the arts and appreciates things of beauty. She is a highly trained dancer who studied classical ballet as a child and young adult, an opera fan who rarely misses a performance at the Metropolitan Opera, a lover of New York City's museums and restaurants, and a writer who composes magazine articles on subjects as diverse as fine wines and kissing.

She got her start in the adult entertainment world as a dancer at Manhattan's world-famous gentlemen's club Scores, where she became quite well known, and even appeared in *The Girls of Scores* movie. She credits radio host and all-around rabble-rouser Howard Stern with putting her on the map. She was invited by producers to participate in a promotion for Stern's radio show, and she thought she would be driving around Manhattan in a bus; she had no idea that she would even meet Howard Stern himself. She arrived at the studio wearing a fur coat with black lingerie underneath, and he was immediately smitten. From their first meeting, Howard Stern was attracted to Savanna not just for her undeniable beauty, but because she is articulate, witty, insightful, and yet humble—in other words, the perfect guest for his radio show. She is a frequent guest on *The Howard Stern Show* and is a favorite of both crew and fans. Whenever Stern held parties at Scores, he always requested that Savanna work that night. Stern was the first to predict she would be very successful in adult movies, and he was right.

Despite her sexy occupation, at first, Savanna had never considered performing in movies. "The more I watched movies, the more I started to get turned on by the idea of doing one myself. I thought, 'I could do that, and I could do that better,' and I wanted to see myself up there on the screen." Her adventurous side came out when she performed in her first adult video in 2000, a European production called *Rocco Meets an American Angel.* She found it to be a liberating and stimulating experience, and before very long, Vivid had her under contract. Reflecting back on her first adult film experience, Savanna says, "That first movie was strangely intimate. It was just Rocco, me, and his cousin with the camera. It was completely different from the types of movies I make now for Vivid, where I have a character and a script. The great sex is incorporated into a story and I love that. It's perfect for me, this kind of work. I love indulging my exhibitionist side, plus the sex is great and I get to act."

Savanna really enjoys working with Vivid director Paul Thomas: "I have a lot of respect for Paul. He knows a lot about acting, and has taught me so much. I was afraid of dialogue and scripts, but I am not anymore and that's because of him—he has this ability to pull something out of me. Plus, he doesn't overdirect me when it comes to the sex; he lets me do my thing." Savanna enjoys her work, and has a movie scene that she considers memorable. "My favorite scene is one with Dale Dabone in *The Wedding.* Our characters were supposed to be reluctant about each other first, and the dynamic and chemistry between us really worked. Then passion took over, and we let loose. The steam from the shower was hot, and we were uninhibited. We did wild things, and it was really fun."

Working for Vivid has had an enormous impact on Savanna's self-image and sexual confidence: "I used to feel guilty about sex; it made me feel like a slut. Now I realize that fantasies are healthy, they are okay. In fact, a lot of my fantasies have a lot to do with stuff I have done on camera first, that I would like to reenact and experience in my real life. Now that I am successful, I have no feelings of regret, no feelings of not wanting to tell people what I do. I have a newfound confidence. My mind continues to open and I am so much more free than I ever was."

Savanna feels that communication is the most important part of a relationship, and a big part of being a better lover. "Once you can master speaking freely about what you like and don't like and are able to express how you are feeling, then everything else falls into place. Don't hesitate to tell your partner about your fantasies," she says. "In my experience, the more open I am, the more receptive my partner is. You can talk about your fantasies during sex, or before actually enacting them. It's also important to be a good listener without judgment."

With a taste for yellow Ferraris and the good life, Savanna has the attitude of a true sexual adventurer. Her number one fantasy locale for having sex is in the Caribbean. "My favorite place in the world is the K Club, a resort in Barbuda, near Antigua. There is amazing white sand everywhere, and nothing else to do but have sex." She also has diverse interests when it comes to sexy background music, which includes Kitaro, Ishamel Lo, Enigma, and African.

Savanna continues to study ballet and theater dance and enjoys going to wine tastings and visiting vineyards in Europe and the United States. She also commutes back and forth from New York City to Southern California to shoot films for Vivid. In addition to her Vivid career, she has had a part in the NBC comedy series *Ed,* posed for a *Vanity Fair* pictorial with famed photographer David LaChapelle, and was the on-scene reporter at the 2003 *AVN* Awards Show for the Metro Channel. *Celebrity Sleuth* magazine chose her as one of "The 25 Sexiest Women in America for 2003." Savanna stays that way by visiting the gym frequently, lifting weights, and doing a rigorous cardio routine.

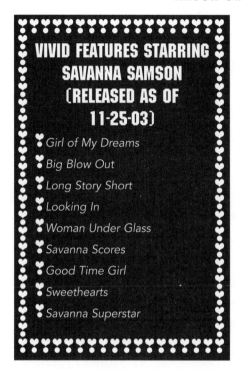

VIVID FEATURES STARRING SAVANNA SAMSON (RELEASED AS OF 11-25-03)

- Girl of My Dreams
- Big Blow Out
- Long Story Short
- Looking In
- Woman Under Glass
- Savanna Scores
- Good Time Girl
- Sweethearts
- Savanna Superstar

SAVANNA SAMSON STATS:

Birthplace: Rochester, NY
Birth date: October 14
Heritage: Italian, Irish, German, Scottish
Measurements: 34C–24–34
Eyes: Brown
Hair: Blondish
Height: 5'5"
Weight: 116
Website: SavannaSamson.com

9
shag tag

Fantasy File:

It's his first professional massage and he eagerly awaits his masseuse. He sits in his briefs on the massage table in the small room, like an eager student on the first day of class. His muscles are slightly sore, but well pumped from an extra-strenuous workout the day before, which he did partly to impress the masseuse. His skin is smooth, shaved that morning as another small attempt to look more attractive to her.

Suddenly the door swings open. In walks a six-foot-tall blonde, long, lean, and toned. She wears six-inch red patent-leather platform boots, matching red patent-leather panties, and a black leather bra fastened with a collar and chains that run from her neck to her waist. The dominatrix looks angry, crazed almost. He jumps slightly at the sight of her, even as he feels his cock tingling with anticipation.

"Lay the fuck down," she commands, her first words to him. "You're smokin'," he tells her, thinking he has paid her a compliment. Displeased that he hasn't obeyed her, she grabs his neck and pushes him down on his back. She walks around the massage table. He asks a question as he stares up at her enormous round breasts, the chains framing them as she struts past. She slaps his face. "Shut up," is all she says. She grabs his feet, roughly pulls his legs out straight, then whacks his thighs with both her hands. The sting from the slap sends a current directly to his cock, and it swells even more, now barely hidden by his underpants.

She walks back to the other end of the table, and stands above his head. Her waist near his face, she climbs up over him, slams his arms down to his side, then pins them down with her knees. Kneeling this way above him, she pulls his dick out with both hands, spits on it, then takes it all the way in to her mouth. Above his face, he sees the swollen lips of her pussy. Hungry to taste her juices, he inhales the musky scent of her arousal and bobs his face up into her. As she licks his giant cock, he laps furiously at her pussy. With each taste of her, he gets more and more aroused, the head of his dick even fatter, the shaft even harder. Releasing his arms from under her knees, he grabs the soft cheeks of her buttocks and kneads them as he slurps away at her. "Eat that pussy," she tells him, this time more of a request than a command. She sits up, then locks both her hands around his dick, and pumps all the way up and down.

Wanting him inside her, she gets up and leans over the side of the small table. Standing behind her, he proceeds to enter her from behind. As soon as he gets inside, it feels so good that he gasps with pleasure. Still leaning forward, she grabs the sides of the table with her hands and braces herself. "Fuck that pussy, bitch!" she yells. He wants to please her, so he does as he's told. "Harder, bitch!" she yells again. With both hands, he grabs onto her waist, then fucks her faster. The table starts to buck and move from the force of his thrusts. She brings one leg up onto the table. He grabs her shoulder and ass as he pumps his dick into her. She grunts like an animal even as she tells him again, "Harder bitch."

He throws his left leg up onto the table, which forces his cock even farther into her. His dick gets so hard he practically lifts her up off the floor as he rams into her from the back. She grunts again. "Fuck me, fuck me." The sweat from his exertion drips off his face onto her back. Now he grabs hold of the sides of the table and rams into her so hard that his feet actually come up off the floor with each thrust. He rotates his hips forward as he drives into her, opening up her hungry wet pussy even farther. The sound of her grunts is accompanied by the loud smacks that peal out each time his groin slams into her ass.

She moves him into a chair, where she sits on his dick. She stays still while he pushes straight up into her, doing it so hard that, again, loud slaps sound out as his thighs smack into her. Next, he sits still as she furiously bobs up and down on his cock. He feels hot, sweaty, almost light-headed from the intensity of her fucking. It's as if all the feeling in his entire body is being drawn into his dick. He feels himself getting closer to coming. With her vast experience, she senses his closeness, then swivels her pussy on his penis to tease him even further. He yells out with pleasure each time she slams back down on his cock. "Fuck me, you bitch," she screams.

Finally satisfied, and knowing that he won't be able to contain himself much longer, she yells at him, "Show me your load, whore." Now standing above her, he takes his dick in his own hand and jerks himself off. As she pushes her breasts together underneath his throbbing cock, he finally lets loose and shoots stream after stream of cum onto her huge tits. His body quivers as it comes out, shaking and twitching with each fresh spurt of jiz. "Oh . . . yes . . . mother . . . fuuuuckerrr," he wails. She slaps him hard across the face. "Don't call me motherfucker," she scolds. "Now get your clothes on and get the fuck out of here."

★★ *from* Good Things,
directed by David Stanley

**" " Sometimes it's cool to just let go of
your inhibitions and go for it. " "**
—*Chi Chi LaRue*

If there's one thing porn stars can be creative with, it's intercourse positions. Of course, some of these are developed more for
camera than for their inherent pleasure, but the stars still manage to
squeeze their bit of pleasure out of each one. With each shift of the
body's position, you stimulate a different area, hit an assortment of hot
spots, and generate varied amounts of friction. The combinations are
seemingly endless, with different variations suiting different moods.

Missionary Positions

**" " Missionary position for me is about
love, romance, and connection. " "**
—*Savanna*

One of the most popular configurations, of course, is the missionary
position, with the woman on her back and the man on top of her. This
allows for lots of kissing, eye contact, and stroking of the breasts and
nipples. Savanna likes this position for the increased level of intimacy it
allows between partners. While "mish," as it's called in the adult movie
world, seems very basic, there are a number of variations you can try
to spice it up. The first is the "knees-up" version: the woman pulls her
knees up toward her shoulders, and the man can lean on her knees or
the backs of her thighs as he thrusts. With her hips tilted upward and
her stomach flattened (a small visual bonus), the woman's clit also angles
up higher. With the woman's knees in between her and her partner, this
leaves room for her to reach down and touch herself as she's being
fucked. Sunrise likes it for the potential G-spot stimulation: "In my private life, my favorite position is missionary with my legs completely up
over my head, or he can use his hands to push my legs down on either

side of me. It just hits me the right way. I never thought it was possible, but if my boyfriend puts me in that position, he hits my G-spot."

In Briana's version, she likes it "when he grabs my ankles and spreads my legs." Yet another "mish" version has the woman wrapping her legs around his thighs, then "locking" her feet under his shins. This provides a little resistance for him to thrust against, and also allows the woman to vary the depth of penetration according to how much she thrusts back. Because both of you are pushing and pulling, this is a particularly high-energy position, but not necessarily tiring, since you are sharing the work. A small drawback is that the in-and-out movement is restricted by the closeness of your bodies. But it's a great way to get started, to look deeply into your partner's eyes, and admire their body as you move together in unison.

Pile Driver and Side Dish

❝ ❝ I like throwing a girl's legs back and fucking her as hard as I can in the missionary [position], all scrunched up. I also like the Reverse Cowgirl and grabbing her thighs and rocking her back and forth on my dick. ❞ ❞

—Bobby

A more gymnastic spin on mish, the Pile Driver can feel really great, and has the added feature of looking totally hot through the camera. Basically, the girl brings her knees all the way up, then swings her feet and legs toward her head. The pelvic tilt makes her pussy face almost straight up, so the motion during intercourse becomes more of an up-and-down piston motion. Guys may need to hang on to her legs to keep them up in the air, and can also use them to brace against during thrusting. The Pile Driver is known for being a great quad workout for the guy, which is why you'll see so many ripped, muscular thighs on the guys in Vivid features. "I always wanted to try the Pile Driver," says Tawny. "I've never done it except in a movie, but I think when people see it in films, they think, 'Hmm, I wonder if I can do that.' A lot of blood rushes to my head and it really does feel good," she adds. In *Chasey Loves Rocco,* a guy and a girl get carried away by lust in the kitchen. Soon she's laid out on the kitchen counter with her knees up and he climbs up and "drives" down into her. Some good rearview camera angles make this movie a good one for Pile Driver pointers.

The Side Dish is an alternate version, where the woman locks her knees together as described in "mish," then rolls over onto her side. If he's got a big rod, you might be able to do it without him sliding out. This happens to be another very camera-friendly position, and also delivers a much different sensation for both partners as the angle of entry changes.

Get a Leg Up—I

Get a Leg Up is also a great position for varied angles of entry and freedom of movement. In this one, the woman lies slightly sideways, with her lower leg extending out, and the other up toward her chest. The guy can be on his knees or standing. In fact, the position works really well when the girl lies on the bed (or table or countertop, wherever) and scoots her rear end to the edge, and the guy stands on the floor. This one also allows lots of room for manual clitoral stimulation, from both the girl and the guy (guys, take a hint!). When doing this one, a lot of guys like to hold on to the girl's up-in-the-air leg, which helps deliver some pretty powerful pushing. In the movies, this is also a favorite since it makes a lot of "slap" between your bodies. In *Good Things,* the pizza deliveryman gets a really big tip when the reformed bitch-on-wheels April offers him her sister to make up for all the mean things she's done to him in the past. During intercourse, the sister Gets a Leg Up while they are both on the bed: she turned slightly sideways with one leg straight up in the air; he on his knees while leaning against her upturned leg. At one point, during slower thrusts, he actually wraps his arms around her leg. At other points, he pushes her leg away and pulls his dick almost all the way out, leaving her begging him to thrust back in. And, yes, there's lots of hot sexy "slap" noises as their bodies slam together, along with some squeaky bedsprings for added ambience. A spin-off move they use in that same scene is "All Together Now," where she is on her back, and he hoists her legs and feet straight up in the air. Holding her legs together creates more friction, which feels good for both partners, and it also tilts up her privates so he can pound her pussy straight on like a ramrod.

Get a Leg Up—II

There's another version of Get a Leg Up to be found in *Good Things.* In this scene, called "Bathroom Buddies," a two-timing Sunrise gets it on in the bathroom of a restaurant with an anonymous guy. At one point, they are both standing up; he enters her from behind as she leans forward with her hands braced against a toilet stall. She turns her body slightly, then lifts one leg all the way up in the air, which he grabs and holds on to. So she stands on one leg, her other up in the air, and he fucks her like a bunny from behind. Because he's slightly taller, he actually goes up and into her with each thrust. The position also allows her lots of room to finger her clit while being fucked; and from the look on her face, she seems pretty pleased.

A related move can be found in *Looking In,* where the nice neighbor lady gets fucked by another neighbor. Here, they both stand up and he fucks her from behind as she leans forward on the table. At one point, she brings one leg up, bent at the knee, and rests it on the table, almost like a sprinter's position. This leaves both his hands free to work on her breasts and clit, and gives her more stability since both her feet are on flat surfaces.

Roly Poly

This is another position in which the girl lies flat on her back. She brings her legs up so that her knees are almost at her ears. Similar to the Pile Driver, this one also tilts her pussy up so that the angle of penetration varies. If the girl is holding her legs up, the guy can massage her breasts and clit. Conversely, if the guy holds the girl's legs in position by pressing against the back of her thighs, this leaves the girl free to do some manual motion on herself. A pillow under the girl's neck will relieve some of the strain on her neck and upper back, while one under her rear end will keep her lower back comfortable. She'll also get a great view of her guy's chiseled chest and shoulder muscles.

Woman on Top

❝❝ I love to be on top. I like to have control of my body, and control of when I am going to come, and I can do that when I'm on top. ❞❞

—*Tawny*

As with the missionary positions, there are several "girl-on-top" positions to choose from. As Tawny notes, the advantage to being on top for women is that they can control the angle of their bodies as well as the depth of penetration. There's also a psychological aspect, as Savanna points out: "I love to be on top when I feel like I want to be in control." Many women like to be on top so that they can move forward and grind against the guy's pubic bone for added clitoral stimulation. "It's easy to come for me with my legs closed and his legs open with me on top. My clit will rub on his pubic bone and make me come really easily," says Briana. The same goes for Kira, although she says this position is almost *too* good for her. "I like being on top, but I get off too quickly," she states. "It only takes a few movements and then there I go; my legs start shaking and it's all over!"

The basic woman-on-top formation has the man on his back, the woman above him resting her knees on either side of the guy. Sitting up straight allows for lots of body massaging as well as an all-access pass to the clit. The woman does most of the movement here, either going up and down or "rocking" forward and back, depending on the type of stimulation she desires. Because you are on your knees, you don't have a ton of room to move around, and sometimes this position doesn't give men enough friction, so it's a good idea to vary the movement from time to time. In *Swoosh,* there are many good examples of this position, both the up-and-down and the rocking version.

Frog Princess

An alternate version involves a woman moving her feet and heels under her and squatting above the guy, instead of resting her knees on the bed. This way a woman's leg muscles can get in on the action, and you piston your entire body up and down. Many women experience a deeper penetration while on top. For some, especially those with extra-large partners, it's too much; but with this position, you can control exactly how far in he goes. Others really like the depth and get very energetic in the up-and-down department. For your guy's sake, be careful not to bounce too much. Sometimes his dick slides out on the upswing, then the girl bounces back down and his hard cock rams into her perineum, and it hurts—a lot! So if it slips out going up, be sure to get it back in before going back down. In *Filthy Rich,* the brunette sister and the lawyer have a hot Frog Princess scene and she does just that. He sits back on the sofa while she squats over him and bounces up and down. When his dick comes out, she is careful to slip him back inside before resuming. The girl adds another little twist to the move, too: she rotates her hips in a circular motion that gives her a break from the vigorous up-and-down motion and also works some other areas of her pussy.

Dasha adds yet another angle to the Frog Princess. "I have one favorite position which doesn't look too good on camera, but I like to do when a guy is lying on his back. I squat and then put my hands on his chest, and lock my knees on my elbows from inside. I look just like a frog, but it's very easy to hold your whole weight that way. You just rock up and down, and it feels really good. You can go as deep as you want to, really slow or really fast, and the guys love it. And you can watch, too. You both get a nice view of everything."

Reverse Cowgirl

Reverse Cowgirl is a position you'll see in many Vivid films, in part because it shows off all the prime parts of a woman's body. For this, the guy is on his back, with his legs either extended out on front of him or hanging off the end of the bed with his feet on the floor. Facing away from his chest, the woman straddles him with her knees bent (if they're both on the bed) or feet on the floor (if his are, too). As with Frog Princess, the woman can bounce up and down or rotate. You'll also see Reverse Cowgirl done with the guy sitting in a low chair, and the girl straddles him backward. Since his penis is entering from a totally different angle, it feels really great for both partners. "I like Reverse Cowgirl and grabbing her thighs and rocking her back and forth," says Bobby. In *Obsession,* the young writer of erotica can't stop thinking about sex. In the first sex scene, he encounters a dancer rehearsing in a studio. At two points, they do Reverse Cowgirl. As he sits on the chair, the lithe dancer squats over his cock with her feet planted on his thighs. This is a perfect position for him to get his hands under her buttocks and help lift them up and down.

Doggie Style

Doggie style is a Vivid Girl favorite. A rear-entry position, it has the woman on all fours with her knees slightly spread apart. The guy can either kneel behind her with his knees together, or stand behind her if she's at the edge of the bed. Doggie style is another position that affords all access to her clit and nipples. For women, if your arms get tired from holding yourself up, try resting on your elbows or even burying your head and shoulders into a pillow. They key is to keep your ass up in the air! Sunrise says: "My favorite position when I am filming is doggie style." Mercedez agreess: "I like doggie style. It gets in deeper. I like to lean down in the front. The angle gets in there really good. I like it with my head on a pillow, but my ass in the air." Mercedez also likes it when the guy squats behind her and they are both on the bed. This move makes for maximal penetration, and guys love the added stimulation.

Briana likes to do doggie at the edge of the bed, with a pillow under her. "You can grind your pussy on the pillow or the edge of the bed, so it's easy to come," she says, adding, "I like looking back and being able to see his dick going in and out." Tawny adds her endorsement of doggie style, too. "It's my favorite position because it hits the right spot. It also gives me the fastest orgasm."

Spoon and Spatula

Spooning is another rear-entry position. Both partners lie on their sides, facing the same direction, with the woman in front. He slips in from behind to penetrate her. This position is all about the angle, and it will vary a lot depending on how long the guy's dick is, if it's curved, and how the girl's vagina is angled. For some folks, there's not enough depth, but the woman bending forward at the waist will alleviate that problem. But, says Briana, "spooning lets me grind against him and get clitoral stimulation that way." It also allows a great deal of full-body contact for your more intimate encounters.

The Spatula is a variant of the Spoon, where the woman lies flat on her stomach. It's a particular fave of Jenna's. "I like to lie on my stomach, totally flat, with my legs together, and have the guy straddle me. My legs are together so I'm able to clench, and there's so much more friction." She also enjoys the same position lying on her back, with the guy on top thrusting between her legs. "It's hard on the guy," she notes, "but it's so good. When you are on your back, you can flex your hips upward and he'll hit your G-spot every time." A good example of spooning is featured in Sunrise's film *Good Things*. April's ex-husband Jack is in bed with his new wife, Diane (Sunrise). After a variety of positions, they settle into a loving spoonful. On their sides, he thrusts slowly and rhythmically into her from behind as he massages her arms, breasts, and stomach and nibbles gently on the back of her neck.

Stand and Deliver

Here's one you've probably seen in many adult movies. The woman stands with her back against a wall or doorway, lifts one knee up (or, if she's really flexible, her whole leg) to expose the good parts. In film plots, this position is always used in hot passionate scenes, where the lovers can't keep their hands off each other. And there is definitely something sexy about a girl just hiking up her skirt to show her guy how much she wants him. Stand and Deliver, of course, works best when the two of you are roughly the same height. For those of different heights (and for really strong guys), here's a Stand and Deliver all-star bonus move. Guys, lift your girl up so her arms wrap around your shoulders and her legs wrap around your waist. Brace your hands underneath her buttocks and then lift her up and down onto your erection. In *Intimate Journey*, one of the couples in the patio sex scene does this, and it's totally hot. The guy's rippled arm and leg muscles work furiously while the girl throws her head back in ecstatic abandon. Gals, try squeezing your muscleman's nipples while in this position, as a little reward for his extra effort.

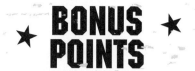

★ **BONUS** ★
POINTS

LOVE TAPS

Guys, one more way to spice up your personal sex profile is to try some love taps. A gentle slap on the rear end during a particularly passionate moment can really rev a girl up. You'll have a nice clear shot in doggie positions and in the missionary 'Leg Up' positions. Keep your fingers together and use your whole open hand to deliver a firm fanny whack right in the middle of her buttock. In films, you'll usually see love taps during supersteamy scenes with lots of hard, fast fucking. In *Obsession*, nice girl-next-door Kira ends up at a wild sex party where she gets it on with three guys at once. It's a pure fantasy scene and the action is hot, intense, and slightly out of control. In this hypersexual scene, it just seems right when one of the guys whacks Kira on the ass. You'll know when it's right for your costar, too.

Yoga Style

Another more intimate, and almost Tantric, position is the yoga move. In this one, the guy and the girl face each other in a seated position and rock back and forth, with the guy's legs extended out underneath the girl's. It requires a fairly large penis, but also allows for lots of kissing, eye contact, and slow touching. For added mobility the guy can lean back on his hands and thrust at a slightly upward angle, which also provides a good view of the action. Or, the woman can snuggle in closer, sit on the guy's thighs, and wrap her legs around his waist. You don't see this position that often in adult movies because, in front of the camera, it looks a little slow and sedate. But in *Good Time Girl,* hot stepmom Savanna finally ends up in bed with her sexy stepson, and they slip into yoga style midway through the action.

The Wave (Motion on the Ocean)

Being strong and flexible is always a plus when performing some of the more acrobatic positions described above. But most of them just require a little practice. Don't forget that penetration doesn't always mean straight in and out. In a hot scene between scheming Dasha and her secret lover in *One Way Out,* the man not only thrusts in and out but moves his hips from side to side as he fucks her. This wavy motion is a great way to vary your technique, and most women love the extra stimulation it affords on their vaginal lips and near their G-spot. Don't be afraid to "borrow" intriguing moves from the movies. Mercedez encourages strongly: "Creative positions are something I've definitely learned from movies. My husband will be trying something different and I'll ask, 'Where did you see that?' and he'll say, 'In a movie!'"

Up Close & Personal
★ Sunrise Adams ★

A true Virgo, soft, innocent, adorable sweetheart Sunrise Adams marks a whole new generation of Vivid Girls. Sunrise is one of the most exciting young talents on the scene, a scrumptiously pretty blonde who just happens to be related to one of the industry's all-time greats. Sunrise is the naughty niece of legendary nineties adult performer Sunset Thomas, from whom she spun off her own stage name. Sunrise loved porn so much she decided to make it her career. "Growing up, I was one of those people watching movies and learning from them," she says. "I still watch movies now. I have the largest porn collection of anyone I know! When my movies are being shot I'm always watching the monitors over the director's shoulder and saying 'Oh yeah, that will look hot.' Even today, if I see a new position I want to try, I use porn to guide me along."

Hers was a fairly boring existence in a town of less than three thousand people in northeast Texas, but Sunrise always found ways to keep herself busy. A slender, well-proportioned beauty, she excels in sports and once played football on her high school team—the first girl ever accepted on the squad. She was also on the track-and-field team, played basketball, rode horses, and played softball on her dad's team.

She found time to amuse herself with other activities as well. "I learned how to masturbate with the water faucet in the bathtub. I progressed on my own from there. I would do it with candles, things I kept hidden in the barn. I had to travel two hours to the closest adult novelty store and an older friend of mine went in and bought me a Pocket Rocket vibrator. I was getting off almost every day." She was also practicing her sexual techniques.

"Sex with my first boyfriend wasn't very good. I never even had an orgasm from sex then. I didn't really enjoy sex until I moved to California and got into the adult industry." She is happy for the opportunities being in adult movies gives her. "I am really learning my body now. I had orgasms when I was growing up, but they were different. With my current boyfriend, I have deeper orgasms because he was the first person to stimulate my G-spot."

She hopes her films will not only expand her sexual

horizons, but those of her fans as well. "I love porn. I love the camera work, I love the lighting, I love taking two people and fulfilling fantasies. Two people expressing themselves sexually? I don't think there is anything negative about it. We're taking people and creating fantasies. We're also creating relationships. When couples have problems, what do they do? They pop in a film and get renewed. They can add to their lives. Maybe you can release something or you can live through that fantasy. We're saving relationships.

"As a viewer, I go for the more romantic stuff. Vivid's films are perfect for me because I love beauty. I hate anything that's disgusting. I don't do choking or a lot of spitting. I like the romantic, really pretty stuff. I do enjoy hard-core close-ups of penetration, but I'm disgusted by the stuff that is degrading. I, and my fans, deserve better." And what is her most memorable movie scene? "My favorite scene is one from *Portrait of Sunrise* I did with Nikita Cash. She was sexy, we both were high energy; it was fun. She just touched all the right places." Sunrise also cites her favorite music for sex as R. Kelly.

Sunrise now lives in the San Fernando Valley, where she raises two puppies: a pit bull and a rottweiler. While she has done and will continue to do mainstream acting, she says, "The adult side of entertainment has always intrigued me and Vivid is an awesome company to work for. They really take care of you like a family. Vivid offers me stability and the ability to grow with them. I want to put as much into the company as they put into me and eventually I'd even like to direct some films."

Meanwhile, Sunrise intends to continue her college education part-time while making films for Vivid. She says she enjoys every minute of adult performing. "The best part of being a porn star is that it is totally positive in its own way. I like knowing that I'm fulfilling people's fantasies and desires, maybe even helping their own romantic relationships."

Sunrise has another talent most women would envy—the ability to size up a man immediately. "I can definitely tell if a man is okay by the way he presents himself. For example, I believe that if he constantly feels the need to walk in front of me, he most likely is going to feel that he's superior to me. Also, it may be old-fashioned but I love the door-opening thing, and I think that whether he displays common courtesy says a lot about how romantic a man will be."

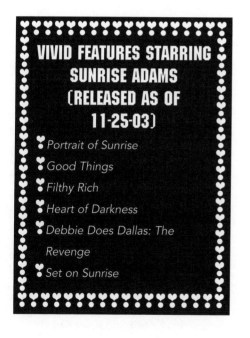

VIVID FEATURES STARRING SUNRISE ADAMS (RELEASED AS OF 11-25-03)

- Portrait of Sunrise
- Good Things
- Filthy Rich
- Heart of Darkness
- Debbie Does Dallas: The Revenge
- Set on Sunrise

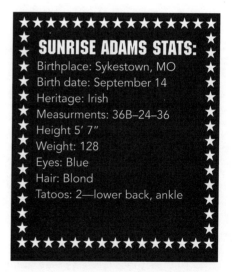

SUNRISE ADAMS STATS:

- Birthplace: Sykestown, MO
- Birth date: September 14
- Heritage: Irish
- Measurments: 36B–24–36
- Height 5' 7"
- Weight: 128
- Eyes: Blue
- Hair: Blond
- Tatoos: 2—lower back, ankle

10
bend over babes and boys

Fantasy File:

The small brunette with large almond-shaped eyes picks up a ripe red strawberry, dips it into a bowl of fresh whipped cream, then puts the whole thing in her mouth, slowly biting it off at the stem. She sits with two enraptured young men, occasionally feeding them cream-topped berries, too. She tells them the story of her first experience with anal sex.

"When I turned twenty-one, my boyfriend at the time wanted to take me to a bar I'd never been to. He took me to this strip bar, and I'd never been to a bar like that. The girls in there were taking their clothes off, real seductively, for all the guys. The guys were going crazy and I started going crazy, too." She takes a long, deep breath as she recalls the evening, then slowly munches on another strawberry. "So then my boyfriend leaned over and he told me, 'When I get you home tonight, I'm going to stick my cock up your ass for your birthday.' So all through the night, I kept thinking about when I got home, how he was going to stick his cock up my ass. He kept reminding me all night that when we got home, that's what he was going to do."

For a moment, her intense gaze fixes upon one of the the young men, who feels a small shiver of excitement run through his body right into his dick. "So we got home and he made sure there was plenty of lube on my ass, plenty of lube, it was just dripping out of my ass. He took the lube and rubbed it all over my asshole, then he pushed some up inside. He put in so much that some of it started to come back out. He told me to lift my butt up, and he slid a pillow under my hips so that my butt stuck straight up in the air at him."

She moans softly, and pauses as she picks up another berry and licks her lips before deciding which young man to feed it to. "I was so anxious at the time, my clit had swollen up like a huge berry." She stops, and dangles the strawberry in front of the young man's eager lips, then continues, "It was as big as this"—referring to the gorgeous ripe berry. "So my pussy got as big as this strawberry; it was absolutely huge. I could feel him getting really close to me, his body getting close to mine. I just about died with excitement. He told me to reach down between my legs and start playing with my clit, so I did."

As she says his, the girl reaches under her dress and starts massaging herself, reenacting her memorable night from years before. "He told me it would loosen my ass up so he could slide his cock into it. So I started playing with it like he told me to. I could feel the head of his cock on the rim of my asshole, then I could feel him start to push it in." She picks up another cream-dipped berry, then rubs it across her nipple, leaving the cream there. One of the young men leans across the table and gently licks it off.

"He went really slow, he started really slow. He didn't want to hurt me. Then he got to the part where the ridge of his head is, the biggest part of his cock, and he made sure he went really slow while he went through that area. Once he got past that area"—she pauses and moans again— "I just sucked his cock right inside of me. He pushed about two or three inches straight in. I just wanted it to go in, so fast. I couldn't wait. He kept easing his way inside me. He kept letting me know how much more cock he had left to go up inside of me, because he said he wanted to feel his balls up against my ass."

She begins unbuckling the pants of one of the young men as she recounts her story. As she opens the guy's fly, she keeps her eyes locked on the other guy sitting opposite. "So he'd tell me, 'You've got three more inches left to put inside of you,' so I'd hold my breath while he put it inside of me. Then he'd say, 'Well, you've got two more inches till I'm all the way inside.' I couldn't wait. I pushed my butt up in the air, and took the rest of it up my ass. I started bouncing up and down. He took his hands and put them on my hips. He pulled me up onto my knees and started fucking me doggie style. He started pulling me into him, fucking me really hard."

She pauses once again, then bucks up as she did for her long-ago boyfriend, letting out a short low gasp. Now totally nude, she grasps the guy's penis. As she does this, the second guy leans forward and caresses and kisses her ass. She leans back into him, resting on his lap as he takes her breasts into his mouth. She continues, "Really hard like he was up inside my pussy. He told me, 'Now don't stop playing with your clit.' So I was just jamming on it, rubbing it really hard while he was fucking me really hard. I couldn't believe it, I had such an orgasm, I had the best orgasm I'd ever had in my life." She rubs her clit now harder, using both hands on herself as she sits on the guy's lap. "I came so hard, it made him come. He shot his hot cum all the way up inside my ass, really deep and really a lot, too. I told him I didn't want him to take his cock out. I told him I wanted to go to sleep with it inside of me. So he pushed it up into me again. I rolled over on my stomach and fell asleep with it inside of me." She leans over, licks her full sensuous lips, and takes the first guy's cock into her mouth, all at once . . .

★★ *from* Intimate Journey,
directed by Judy Blue

Anal Sex

Some of the most popular adult titles today are anal sex videos, with a number of Vivid films featuring it. Anal pleasure is an often-misunderstood area of sexuality, tinged with fear, shame, and anxiety. When done correctly, though, it can be an extraordinarily intimate, intense experience for both partners. Many of the players on Team Vivid rave about backdoor sex, while others are just beginning to test it out. No matter what their level of experience, though, everyone has something to say about it.

Anal 101

❝❝I am so removed from anal sex in films, but I really enjoy anal sex privately. For me, it's more of a giving something to the person I love. It's not something I could do with a man the first time. I have to be in love with him. ❞❞

—Jenna

"When I was a dancer at Scores, men would tell their fantasies, and they all wanted to have anal sex, but their wives or girlfriends wouldn't give it up," says Savanna. She points out a pretty common scenario: men who want to give anal a try and their female partners who say "no way." Many women resist anal sex based on a number of assumptions that are often untrue. Many people assume that it's dirty, painful, and dangerous, along with other connotations such as guys who like it are gay, or that's it's a very high-risk activity. The fact is that when done properly, anal sex can not only be pain-free, but very pleasurable. And with good hygiene and condoms, it won't be messy or risky.

The anus, anal canal, and rectum are made of tissue that is very rich in nerve endings, and very responsive to stimulation, vibration, and penetration. Many women experience indirect G-spot stimulation through anal penetration and a number of them say that anal sex can lead to amazing orgasms. Savanna likes to combine anal with clitoral stimulation, and puts it a little more bluntly: "I use a vibrator on my clit during anal sex. For me, a vibe on the clit plus a dick in the ass equals a great orgasm." So there you go.

Beyond the physical pleasures, the psychological aspects of anal sex also make it appealing to some people. The idea that it's naughty and taboo, and that "nice" girls don't do it, can heighten the erotic experience. For Jenna, anal is a unique and relatively rare occurrence. The fact that it's special adds to the pleasure of her experience. "You have to trust your partner to not hurt you. I've noticed that when I'm in love with a person . . . it gets me off knowing that he's the only man getting it," she states.

Trust and communication are important in all kinds of sex, but they are essential with anal sex. You are dealing with a very delicate part of the body, so you must trust your partner completely. Sunrise is just beginning to explore anal action: "You have to find the right person who you feel safe and secure enough to do it with. If you find that person, you can let that 'secret part' of you go," she says. "Slowly, I am working to achieve that. It's definitely a work in progress." Talking is crucial: the receptive partner should be very clear about slow or fast they like it, how deep or not so deep, and when they are ready for the next step.

Before getting into specifics, you need to know about prep work. For film shoots, the stars always have an enema before filming. However, this is not absolutely necessary for clean anal sex; often going to the bathroom followed by a thorough shower is enough to ensure a comfortable experience for both partners. If you are nervous about being squeaky-clean, and know in advance that you will be doing it, then an enema is advisable several hours before the hot date. You don't want to do it right before sex, because the body needs some recovery time. The porn-star rule of thumb is: enema the night before a morning shoot, and an A.M. enema for an evening one. You can use a prepackaged enema from the pharmacy and just follow the simple directions on the package. Since you'll be using it for sex and not for digestive problems, some stars recommend emptying out the store-bought solution and using just plain water.

Backdoor Basics

" " **My biggest tip is just relax. If you don't like doing it, then don't do it. After the first time, I wasn't scared anymore and I was able to experiment and get more creative.** " "

—*Briana*

As Briana notes, relaxation is essential for good anal sex. Taking deep, slow breaths and being sexually aroused will kick off the relaxation process. "My first anal scene was in *The Watcher*. It was supposed to be a three-way with Bobby and Pat; they just kind of talked me into doing it anal. It hurt that first time. Bobby [is] very well endowed and went really slow, but I don't think I got off on it that time. After that, I wasn't scared to try it, though. I was able to experiment more and get more creative. There are so many ways you can do it."

The more aroused you are, the likelier it is that you will enjoy anal penetration, so plenty of foreplay is advised. Tawny, whose anal adventures occur more offscreen than on these days, says, "I learned to like anal sex, but I didn't start out that way. I was nervous and convinced it would hurt. Now I know I can relax. My ass can open up with lots of foreplay."

Sunrise likes to start with simple external stimulation. "I have only had anal sex on film a few times. In my private life, I am experimenting with it. It can be a scary thing: that's a very sensitive part of the body and you really have to take your time. I like it when my partner rubs his fingers just on the outside of my asshole. I like to go slow, really take our time." Mercedez uses a slightly different approach: "If I am going to do any kind of anal, I have to have a vibrator to get my mind off it in the beginning."

Jenna likes a guy to go in and stay there until she gets used to the feeling. "He has to have a really good hard-on, because he has to inch his way in," she says. "Once he gets all the way in, I have to have him sit there for a couple of minutes to be able to get used to it. Once I'm used to it, he can slowly start stroking, but not all the way out. It's so hot, it really is hot. It seems like a no-no, but it's a once-in-every-three-months kind of thing—and I have to have a glass of wine."

In *Jenna Loves Rocco,* there's a steamy three-way scene between a guy and two girls in dominatrix outfits. After much foreplay and vaginal penetration, the guy begins anal penetration of one of the girls as she lies on her stomach. Prelubricated, he rubs his dick up and down the crack of her ass to help stimulate the area. First, he slides in just the head, and then waits a bit before going any farther. This is a great tip for guys: go in a little bit at a time, which gives the girl's muscles a chance to adjust. In the film, he enters bit by bit and, a few minutes later, proceeds to a faster and harder pace in a doggie-style position.

Analingus, also called rimming, is another great way to begin your anal explorations. As Chi Chi explains: "I'm big on rimming, which you don't see in a lot of straight porn movies. The ass is a very big erogenous zone that isn't explored by a lot of heterosexual couples. I've been doing it in all my Vivid movies and the results are incredibly hot." He adds, "Make sure everything is nice and clean for your partner. It's kind of fun, dirty and sexy, and maybe takes you to a nastier place without it being too nasty." Rimming can be done around the outside of the asshole; you can also use your tongue to penetrate just inside the hole. In the very first sex scene of *Where the Boys Aren't 15,* Dasha gets a hot rim job from one of the other girls. In the back of a van, the brunette throws Dasha's legs up in the air, spits on her hole, and then tongue-fucks her in the rear end. Her pierced tongue only adds to the pleasure. She also lubes up her fingers with spit, and massages all around Dasha's entire anal area. All of which adds up to the perfect prelude for anal penetration.

Another essential prep move is having lots of lube on hand. Unlike the vagina, the ass is not self-lubricating, so you'll need some outside assistance. In this case, spit usually just won't cut it. Jenna, on the other hand, prefers saliva because she says some lubes can sting. Guys take note: lack of lube is probably the number one reason why women are turned off by anal. Do it right, and you'll be doing it often. Savanna says, "You can't do it without lube. Lube makes penetration easier it makes it feel better." Thicker lubricants are great for anal sex since they stay wet longer and have a cushioning effect on the delicate tissue inside the ass. For more specifics on lube types and brands, see Chapter 7. And remember, there's no such thing as too much lube when it comes to someone's ass, so don't be stingy!

The second biggest mistake guys make when it comes to anal is going too fast. The rectum needs slow, patient, gentle exploration to get it relaxed enough for penetration. When you start to enter, many women like clitoral or vaginal stimulation at the same time to help ease the big entrance. "I really love it when a man's going down on me to use his fingers in my ass, but I usually have to ask for it," says Savanna. For Sunrise, her vibrator is the key to good anal action. "I use lots of lube and I like to have the Pocket Rocket on my clit and another vibrator right on the outside of my vagina. When all the parts are stimulated, penetration is much easier for me," she notes.

A great way to warm up is to slowly build up. Start with your fingers or a small toy. Here's Dasha's advice: "I enjoy anal sex only with someone who knows how to do it right, and only in certain positions, so I do it mostly with my husband. He's had a chance to find out how to do it, and what feels best for me. Some girls can relax and open up right away, but I'm not like that. You have to stimulate that area first, then use fingers, to get that area ready; sometimes I do it myself. It usually hurts a little bit at the beginning, but once it gets stretched, it feels amazing."

Once you have warmed her up, and she seems ready for more, you still need to go slowly as you penetrate her. "I think what's important to remember about anal sex is that women are afraid it will hurt. The first time the idea is to put it in slightly, take it out, and then try it again. Maybe it'll take three times until it feels right. But what happens is, as the muscles dilate, then it goes in easier and it feels great," advises Savanna.

Preferred Positions

It's important to experiment with different positions to find which ones work best for you. Savanna's favorites? "If you're doing it for the first time, then try the spoon position, or in missionary position. I love anal sex in the missionary position, but my favorite for anal is spooning with the man behind me," she states. Savanna also steers novices away from another popular position. "Doggie style is not going to be good for the girl. Later, when she's all completely relaxed, then yeah, bend over and do it. But I recommend other positions to start. Don't expect to be on all fours and feeling good until you get used to it."

Dasha feels the same. "Even though I love anal, and I do so much with it, it hurts me doggie style. The best for me is missionary, sometimes spooning, lying on our sides with the guy behind me. I have a type of orgasm that I've never had before; every hair on my head [is] tingling and it [is] like a shock throughout my whole body. So once you get through the first ten seconds—try to get through it—it feels really good. You just have to discover the right position."

Advanced Anal

❝❝I like anal penetration. Straight up, it makes me come. I found out I was multiorgasmic when I tried anal sex. I had no idea I would like it until I finally did it. ❞❞

—*Kira*

Kira considers anal one of her on-screen specialties, and confesses that it's also one of her favorites offscreen. Like Dasha and Savanna, she recommends some warm-up exercises: "If I'm on top, then I like to stick a couple of fingers in my ass. If he's doing me from behind, I like it when he busts out a dildo or vibrator. Just relax, because if you tense up, it's going to hurt."

For advanced anal, you might want to try double penetration. It not only makes for a hot visual on film, but also gets all her parts in on the action. "Double penetration takes me beyond the stars as far as orgasm is concerned," Kira says. "It's mind-blowing." Kira has double-penetration scenes in *Nurses,* and also in *Obsession.* In *Nurses,* Kira plays Nurse Tang, who is recruited by her psychiatrist boss to have some major three-way anal action with two doctors in order to test if his behavior modification experiment has worked on a sex pervert. That film has some superhot ass licking, ass fucking, and, in another scene, some ass fucking in a sling. In *Obsession,* Kira gets it on with three guys in a group scene, and the double penetration occurs after warm up stints with both vaginal and anal. Toward the end, she takes them both. The usual position is that one guy lies flat on his back, with the girl facing him and sitting on his dick. The second guy comes in from the rear, and usually squats or goes into a push-up position as he penetrates her ass. This is also how Dasha does it in the locker room scene with the two football jocks in *Student Body.* Whether you decide to do double or not, it's definitely fantasy material.

Finally, one new trend in adult movies that used to be strictly forbidden is men experiencing anal pleasure. Chi Chi is at the forefront of this innovation and describes an experience he recently had on the set. "Dale Dabone had never done anything anal on film. In a film I was directing, he was working with Lola, a girl who really loves making a scene. Lola went to rub his ass, and at first he said he didn't want her to because he thought if he got his ass played with, it would look gay. I told him, 'It's not gay if a girl is doing it to you.' He went for it and loved it." Chi Chi makes an important point: getting off on anal play does not make a guy gay. All the points we discussed during anal anatomy and pleasure can apply to both women and men. Plus, men have the prostate gland, which can be stimulated through anal penetration and feels pretty good. Women may want to explore the possibility, even if their guy isn't quite ready for them to strap on a dildo. "If a woman is giving a man a blow job, nibbling on his balls, she can sneak a little tongue in there," Chi Chi advises. "A lot of guys would be receptive; you'd be surprised. If a guy is getting ready to ejaculate, putting a finger up his butt can really increase his pleasure. He just has to be receptive to it."

Up Close & Personal
★ Tawny Roberts ★

Born in Utah and raised in Dallas, Tawny was a basketball, volleyball, and golf star in high school. She studied retail management in college and, after graduation, entered the management training program at a Los Angeles department store, where she worked in the lingerie department. A few years ago, renowned performer/director Jill Kelly and former Dayton Rains approached Tawny at a Hollywood nightclub, and asked her if she'd ever considered performing in adult movies. "They told me a lot about the adult industry, and their own experiences as performers. It sounded really positive—not what I expected. I got in touch with Dayton, and she introduced me to some photographers. My first magazine layout was a pictorial with Dayton in *Hustler* magazine in January 2002."

Tawny had only ever seen a handful of porn movies, and never imagined she could have sex on film. But she decided to give it a shot. She was cast by Jill Kelly in a film called *Immortals.* "I was incredibly nervous. I remember that there was a script, and I had some dialogue. I memorized it, but when we started shooting, I kept forgetting my lines! The sex part was easier, because I knew my male costar, Rick Patrick. I felt comfortable with him. Then Jill put me in touch with Jim South and World Modeling, and very soon after, my movie career took off."

Her career has changed her perception of the much-maligned industry. "Before I was in the industry, I didn't think highly of porn stars. They were always portrayed as sexual freaks, drug addicts, and sluts. Now I know they are normal people, more normal than you think. I've made a lot of good friends in the business, and I have so much respect for women in porn. It's better than I ever imagined it would be."

Being part of the adult entertainment world has had a very positive effect on Tawny's life. "I grew up in a conservative, religious family. I was extremely sexually repressed. In fact, I didn't consider myself sexual before I got into the industry. Working in adult movies has opened my eyes and my mind to so many new things. I used to be very shy about everything; now I am ready to try new things all the time. In order to be good at my job, I have really had to figure out what feels good, learn my body and what turns me on, and be open to experiencing new things," says the lusty blonde. "I did my first scene with another woman on camera, and it changed my life. I discovered I am really attracted to girls, and I love having sex with them." And what was Tawny's most memorable on-camera scene? "Doing a scene with Jenna Jameson for her website was the best; I was really attracted to her, we both used strap-ons on each other, and I fulfilled one of my ultimate fantasies. I don't know if I would have had an opportunity to explore that side of myself if I wasn't in porn."

Tawny says she prefers having someone undress her to undressing herself. "I like to have someone take control; I like for people to do things to me." True Pisces that she is, one of Tawny's erogenous zones is her feet. "I like my toes sucked; it feels really good. I have it done in private and on film. It's an awesome feeling and it's different." Her choice of music for sex? "It depends on my mood. If I've been out partying I like techno, hip-hop, and Eminem."

With more than thirty adult movies under her belt, Tawny is a rising star, known for her enthusiasm and her amazing body, which comes from her love of sports: "I'm a pretty normal girl who loves my work," says Tawny. "I have a full life and am active all the time. I love to run, work out, hit the slopes with my snowboard, play a few rounds of golf, or go wakeboarding with my friends. I exercise all the time. I love to travel and do it as much [of it] as I can." Two of her favorites places are Las Vegas and Cancún, Mexico. In fact, the beach is her favorite sexy hot spot. "I think the beach is incredibly romantic. A long walk in the sand followed by sex is really wonderful. The water is there, so you can have sex in the water, too."

In addition to all the traveling she does for feature dancing, film locations, and promotional events, Tawny's favorite part of her job is her fans: "I like the attention from fans, I love to do signings and events where I get to meet them. When fans tell me what their favorite movie of mine is or a favorite scene they loved, it really gets me excited. It turns me on that people are watching me have sex and getting turned on."

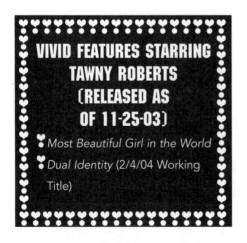

VIVID FEATURES STARRING TAWNY ROBERTS (RELEASED AS OF 11-25-03)

♥ *Most Beautiful Girl in the World*

♥ *Dual Identity* (2/4/04 Working Title)

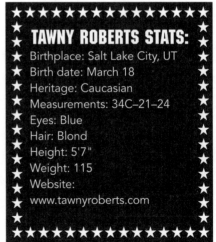

TAWNY ROBERTS STATS:

★ Birthplace: Salt Lake City, UT
★ Birth date: March 18
★ Heritage: Caucasian
★ Measurements: 34C–21–24
★ Eyes: Blue
★ Hair: Blond
★ Height: 5'7"
★ Weight: 115
★ Website:
www.tawnyroberts.com

11
the money shot

Fantasy File:

When she received the subtly worded invitation to the "party," she had no idea it would be like this. Room after room of people in leather and bondage gear, people in slings and tied up, and doing things she had only imagined. They led her inside and she changed into a patent-leather bustier with a collar around her neck and thigh-high leather boots with stiletto heels. She could feel the sexual energy in the air, and it excited her. She finds herself in a room with three men at once. Each one is muscular and lean, with six-pack abs, like guys she had only seen in magazines. One by one, the guys strip off their clothes, revealing huge perfectly shaped cocks that bolt straight up in their hardness.

Just looking at them, she feels her skin tingle and her thighs tense up with anticipation. She sits on the floor and the three guys surround her, stroking their cocks. They're all so hot, almost instinctively, she opens her mouth to take in the first guy. She puts as much of it as she can in her mouth, all the while watching the other two guys still stroking themselves. She stands and bends forward so she can taste the second guy. While she does this, a bolt of electricity flies through her body when the first guy inserts his finger into her aching hole. Her lips uncontrollably pull his finger up inside her. She's never felt so free to explore her own sexuality, and she keeps moving from one guy to the next so she can savor as much of the experience as possible. The first one massages her ass, a second her breasts. Her entire body seems to cry out for more.

Finally he begins fucking her from behind. She's never felt such a huge dick inside her before, and every inch of it fills her with passion. He holds on to her hips as he rides her faster and harder. Meanwhile the second guy puts his cock in her mouth. With each thrust from behind, she finds herself taking more of the second guy's cock into her mouth. Next, she sits on the second man's dick while he lies on the floor. She rides him so hard that her butt cheeks slap against his hips each time she comes down. She decides she wants to do it all. She rolls over on her back and tells him to fuck her in the ass. He applies some lube to her and she feels her muscles loosening up. He enters slowly. "That's it, baby, you want it up there, don't you?" he asks in a deep husky voice. "Yes, yes" is all she can think to say. Soon, the thought occurs to her. If not now, when? She wants two guys inside her at once. The third guy lies on the floor and she sits on his dick while the second guy comes up behind her and continues his penetration of her ass. She feels herself losing control of her own body as every pore and muscle seem to quiver with sexual excitement.

She reaches down to touch her clit, and seconds later, it hits her. Her whole body starts tingling and shaking; she never in her wildest fantasies imagined she could feel this way. Wave after wave of sheer ecstasy starts in her vagina and ripples through her entire body like a tidal wave. She feels each one hit until she can't take anymore. She sits on the floor surrounded by her three dream lovers. Now they are ready, too. She watches them closely as they stroke themselves into their own climaxes. The first strokes slowly and holds just the shaft; the second applies more lube and strokes quickly, focusing on just the head; the third stays off to the side and slowly moves his hand up and down his entire cock. The first guy quickens his pace and shoots across her breasts. The second places his thumb behind the head of his cock and strokes rapidly, then he, too, shoots load upon load of creamy jiz onto her neck and chest. She climbs over to third guy and takes his dick in her mouth one more time. Finally ready to explode, he takes his cock into his own hands and strokes all the way up and down. He stops for just a second, tightly gripping his cock just below the ridge of the head, then lets out a big stream of cum that shoots across to her, covering her yet again. Still drawn to his gorgeous body and handsome face, she wonders for a second if this all really happened, or if it was just a dream.

★★ *from* Obsession,
directed by Paul Thomas

All About Orgasms

If you've watched an adult movie lately, it will come as no surprise that the sex scenes often last for twenty minutes or more, and that's after editing down from two hours of footage. In fact, the thing that most people, especially men, probably envy most about porn stars is their staying power. This doesn't mean that good sex always has to take hours, since we all know a quickie can be pretty good, too. But if you want to know how to keep the fire burning longer, or how to delay your orgasm to make it more intense, then let the porn stars be your guide. The so-called money shot has always been a necessary one in adult movies. These days, you're as likely to see women come on camera as men. In this chapter, Team Vivid tells you all about orgasms and some ways to achieve your ultimate sexual satisfaction.

Making It Last

One thing we've noted several times is that the more time you spend *reaching* an orgasm, the more time you'll spend *having* an orgasm. Actors often need to draw out a scene so the director can have plenty of footage to work with, so here are some star-tested techniques for making it last. The first, of course, is to spend lots of time on foreplay. This includes everything from kissing and massage to hand jobs, oral action, and sex toys. Not only does this extend your encounter, but it also builds the tension between the two of you, heightens your arousal, and makes use of the all-important tease we've talked about in so many other sections. Jenna's ideal encounter: "It's a slow buildup that does it for me. It's more of a teasing thing; the slower someone goes, the better. I could probably come in like five minutes, but if a guy is well trained in the art of teasing, then after a half hour or forty-five minutes, when I do come, that's the best, the most intense."

For men, once you've begun intercourse, try this: slow down, stroke more slowly, and reduce the pace. This works for some, but others still find it too stimulating. To bring it down another notch, try lying still with your cock inside her, but don't move your hips. The motion of her breathing and the clenching of her muscles will be the only stimuli on your dick. Shift your attention away from your penis. Kiss her neck, caress her body, but don't thrust in or out.

For some, just the feel of her vaginal muscles is enough to put them over the top. If you find yourself in this position, and you want to put off your orgasm, then it's time to pull out completely and take a little breather. "Tease the guy, switch positions," advises Tawny. "It will break the momentum and make it last." Some recommended activities during your time-out: licking her pussy to build up her anticipation even further, and switching positions to alter the rhythm and intensity. This method can work for women, too. Kira notes, "I've stopped myself from coming a lot of times. [I] break the rhythm and then get started again, because I want it to last longer. I get a bigger orgasm out of it."

Jenna suggests that men also become aware of their arousal patterns and practice delaying ejaculation. "I think a lot of that is the man's duty to practice when he's masturbating, to be able to know when he's about to come. Maybe pull out and go down on the girl so he doesn't end up coming. If we haven't had sex in a while, my partner's constantly pulling out. You have to know your own body really well." And on those occasions when it just happens before you want it to? "Just wait fifteen minutes and do it again!" Jenna suggests.

Paul Thomas is a big fan of really drawing out the process, sometimes for days. He feels that just because you've begun to have intercourse, there's no reason you can't stop, change activities, or even stop having sex for a while and begin again later. "What's really satisfying is when I'm with the woman I'm with now. I'll watch her getting dressed in the morning and we may tweak and suck a little here and there, begin on Friday, and not even have an orgasm until Sunday. I'm in this horny state of bliss all weekend."

The Big O

❝ ❝ An orgasm is like a series of waves. Whenever you watch a guy come you see him go squirt, squirt. It's the same for the girl really. Every muscle's flexing, it's like the most amazing thing in the world. ❞ ❞

—*Jenna*

Ask twenty people how they like to achieve an orgasm, and you're sure to get twenty different answers. The preferred method of getting there, when they climax, how many times, and how important an orgasm is to their overall satisfaction all vary from one person to the next. Some men, for example, like to come during intercourse, while others prefer a blow job or manual action. In films, the money shot must be seen by the camera, so most male actors stop intercourse and ejaculate somewhere on the woman's body. Chi Chi likes it when both actors are involved in the money shot. "If someone jacks somebody off, visually it's really great. If someone can bring someone else to a climax, that's more appealing than someone doing it to himself. I always try to get the girl to finish him off. It seems hotter that she can make him come."

Indeed, most men would agree that it's nice to have a hand other than their own bring them to orgasm. One trick that Mercedez learned involves inviting the balls to the party. "I worked with a guy who told me to stroke his balls as he was about to come. So I started to do that to others, and it can really send a man over the edge." Some guys have very specific techniques for making themselves come, though, and often prefer to do it themselves. In his films, Bobby strokes so quickly just before coming that it looks like the video is on fast-forward. Some guys just rub the head with their whole hand, some go all the way up and down the shaft, and some do the hand twist. Most like a faster and tighter grip as they approach orgasm. As we noted in Chapter 8, it's always a good idea to watch how a guy strokes himself, then try to duplicate it back on him.

As countless men's-magazine articles will attest, women have a reputation for being more complicated in the climax department. For starters, some women are just more naturally orgasmic than others. They can come from oral sex, clitoral stimulation, vaginal penetration, G-spot stimulation, anal penetration, or any combination of these. Jenna's one of the versatile women who enjoys something inside or outside. "Penetration alone or external clit stimulation alone can make me come. They're both so incredible. With penetration, my orgasm is so much different; it's more work for the guy, but the orgasm for me is better. It's definitely easier for me to come from having my clit stimulated."

The Vivid Girls as a group embrace a wide variety of stimuli, although almost like clitoral stimulation to be at least one part of the mix. Sunrise says, "The easiest way for me to have an orgasm is to be in Reverse Cowgirl position for vaginal penetration, and not have him all the way inside. Plus, a Pocket Rocket on my clit." Mercedez also says a vibrator on her clit is the easiest way for her to come. Briana and Kira are fans of the anal way. Briana's preferred position: "On my stomach, rubbing my clit against a pillow and having my ass penetrated." As we noted in Chapter 10, Kira likes anal penetration "straight up" for coming and multiple orgasms. Savanna prefers just a little bit of anal excitement during her climax. "I love it when I have a mouth on my clit and then a finger in my ass. That gives me an orgasm right away," she says. For Tawny, vaginal penetration alone in the doggie position works, or "if I have sex with a woman, I like oral sex and some fingers. That makes me comes fast," she confesses.

The majority of women, porn star or not, rank clitoral stimulation as their number one orgasm inducer, whether with a hand, a tongue, or a vibrator. Whatever your preference, it's important to communicate with your partner. And, in the same way that women can watch and learn how their guy likes to come, it's good idea for women not only to tell, but to show, their partners some of their own masturbation techniques. As Jenna notes, "Sure I can make myself come. But it's so much better when someone else gives you an orgasm. It's almost surprising when someone else can do it."

Multiples

❝ ❝ When I am masturbating, in ten minutes, I can have five, six, seven orgasms easily. ❞ ❞

—Dasha

Like Dasha, women can experience multiple orgasms when they masturbate alone or during sex with a partner. Tawny discovered her multiorgasmic ability while working in adult movies. "I can definitely come a lot more than just once. In the industry, I am having sex for so long on a shoot that it's inevitable. But I recover quickly and just keep going," she says. For Mercedez, multiples are more likely to occur at home than on the set, depending on how relaxed she is and the level of intimacy she has with her partner. "If the sex is really good, I can have multiple orgasms," she says. "With my partner, I am totally relaxed, uninhibited. When there's nothing in the back of my mind, I'm not worried about anything. I can let go and keep going."

Some multiorgasmic women need a brief period of downtime. Then, once their body recovers, they can continue. Others don't have to wait until one subsides before they start building up for the next. It's possible to intensify the sensation from one to the next by overlapping them. Kira experiences orgasms both ways, depending on the activity. "My orgasms definitely build on one another. For me, that's mostly with anal sex. If it's vaginal penetration, I can definitely feel the difference, the orgasms feel more separate. But with anal sex, they just come one right after another." In either case, though, most women report that their clitoris is too sensitive to be touched right after orgasm. So men should stimulate other areas until she's ready for more. Other women like a guy to stop for fifteen to thirty seconds after she's come, then start rubbing her clit again, stopping and starting like this for as many times she feels she can come—which could be as many as a dozen times. Still other women prefer to stop stimulation of the area altogether for a while, and like to switch from vaginal penetration to anal, or from anal to oral.

For Dasha, coming once or in multiples depends on what she's doing. Clitoral stimulation, whether from her own hand or a partner's, is her surefire way to get there. "When I do it myself, I lie on my belly and play with my clitoris and I can come six or seven times in a short period. When a guy works my clit with his hands, I can have multiples, too. It's not that easy with just intercourse. When I have my clit stimulated during intercourse, it makes the sensation more intense, but it seems to take attention away from just focusing on my clitoris. Intercourse with clitoral stimulation feels better, but it doesn't make me have as many orgasms," she points out.

Briana says she can come many times, but prefers not to. "I like to get real close to coming, then go back to kissing and touching. I'll say, 'Pull it out, pull it out.' I like to save it up and have one huge orgasm. I have the ability to have lots of little ones, but I like to save it up," she says. Similarly, Savanna is a devotee of the save-it school. "I've had a couple of orgasms in one session. The most I've had is three, but that's rare. I have one big one and then I'm done. In my private life, if we are going to have anal sex, I don't like to have an orgasm until we get there, because the orgasm is so much more intense. So I delay it, then once I have something in my ass, I go for the big one."

She Squirts

❝ I think one of the most amazing things I ever saw was Dasha's squirting orgasms. Dasha had this amazing squirting orgasm and Jenna turned to the camera and said, 'Did you get that?' ❞

—Chi Chi

If you've seen Dasha's infamous squirting orgasms on-screen or had sex with someone who had them, then you know that some women can ejaculate. Those who do usually ejaculate from direct G-spot stimulation. As the G-spot is stimulated, the paraurethral glands produce fluid, which is released through the urethra. Because it comes out the same opening as urine, some people mistakenly think the girl is peeing, but she is actually ejaculating. Research shows that female ejaculatory fluid has a different chemical makeup than urine; the fluid is usually thin and clear and smells sweet. Because of that, female ejaculation is tough to capture on film, and it is usually shown in slow motion. In *Student Body*, when Dasha goes to the professor for some extra credit, she shoots. She lies back on the professor's desk while he goes for her G-spot with his fingers. The camera pans back a bit to get it on film.

Among the Vivid Girls, Dasha is the most experienced squirter. But it wasn't until she started making films that she realized not all women do it. "When I was younger, I did it with my longtime boyfriend, and he really liked it. But I had no idea that only a few people could do it," she says. It's easiest for her to ejaculate from someone stimulating her G-spot with their fingers, as the professor does in *Student Body*. Although she squirts fairly easily, it doesn't happen every time. "I do it whenever I feel like it. Often a director asks me, 'Can you do it right now?' But it doesn't work that way. Sometimes my body's not in the mood, especially if I am dehydrated. Generally, though, if it's really passionate and the guy is really excited about the scene, then it works."

Kira's also a squirter, but she does it during intercourse rather than through manual stimulation. "I experienced it the very first time just by playing with a sex toy. I got off five times, then all of a sudden I soaked the bed. I thought I peed, but I didn't. A lot of women can squirt and just don't know it. I ejaculate once in a while, but it takes a lot out of me." Kira also notes that it doesn't happen every time. When it does, she says, she has to have already come a few times and she has to be on top. "I know when I'm going to squirt because I get that feeling like when a sponge fills up with water. You just want to squirt it out. It's such a powerful urge. I get so light-headed right after," she relates.

Vigorous, consistent G-spot stimulation is the best way to achieve ejaculation. Most women report that they feel as though they have to pee before they ejaculate. If, instead of tensing up, she relaxes and bears down, she can often ejaculate. Kira learned her preferred technique on the Vivid set: "A lot of guys in the business started cupping their fingers once they were inside. Angling the fingers, or using toys that are curved, hits my G-spot and makes me squirt instantly," she explains.

Sunrise's preferred position is different from either Dasha's or Kira's. "If I get into the missionary position, then put my legs completely up over my head into Pile Driver, he just hits me the right way. If my boyfriend puts me in that position, he hits my G-spot and I can gush," Sunrise explains, adding that she can only do it at home, not on film. The Vivid Team says that doggie style is another good position for squirting, with your head and shoulders down and your bot-

tom up. This angles your body perfectly, so that when you are penetrated, your partner can't miss your G-spot.

Timing

Romance novels would have you believe that simultaneous orgasms
are both very common and the culmination of some deep romantic
attachment. The truth is that it's more of an ideal than a reality. It's
nice if it happens, but you certainly shouldn't be disappointed if it
doesn't. Paul notes that there is a certain amount of compromise in
the whole who-goes-first thing when it comes to orgasms. "No one
person has more virtue than the other. The one who is ready to stop
has to be ready to continue and the one who wants to continue has to
be ready to stop. It has to be. An orgasm, like sex, is not something
that should be forced. If one partner is really ready to stop, then the
other has to respect that."

In adult movies, you won't see simultaneous orgasms, since the
money shot has to be visible and come last, and not during intercourse. But since your own adventures probably take place off camera, you might want to give it a try. Simultaneous orgasms don't
happen by magic, or because of true love. The simple fact is that one
person has to hold back until the other is ready, and then let loose.
This requires knowing your body well, communicating to your partner how close you are, so you can synchronize. Again, don't be dis-
mayed if you try and miss. As Dasha notes, "It's no big deal if it
doesn't happen. Definitely when it's possible, it's great, but it's not always easy to coordinate."

Savanna offers some specific tips on making it happen. You have
to have good awareness of your body and control over when you
come, both of which will happen with practice. "I love coming simultaneously," she states. "It's very easy for me to come, so the second the guy says, 'I'm going to come,' it's easy for me to do it at the
same time. If I'm having two, it's usually when he says he's going to
come I have my second one." Since men generally have an easier time
climaxing than women, it is usually they who have to delay. When the

woman lets him know that she's close, he can concentrate on coming at the same time.

Target Practice

Another thing you might have noticed in adult movies lately is that the guys don't always shoot their loads on the girl's stomach. While there's certainly a lot of coming onto breasts or the neck and face, we've also been seeing guys coming on the girls' feet. Chi Chi also notes that in the business, when a guy comes on a woman's face, it's called a "facial." In *One Way Out,* when Dasha has sex with her obnoxious husband, he shoots his load all over her pretty manicured feet. In that film, it happens in a couple of other scenes as well.

For guys, it's not just about hitting a particular target. Distance is another thing they get off on. In *Looking In,* the swinging neighbors have sex in the living room. When the guy is ready to come, he hauls back and shoots his load several feet into the air. It's quite a sight to behold. In addition to distance, volume is another factor. In *Intimate Journey,* during the group-sex-on-the-patio scene, the guy who fucks the spiky-haired blonde unleashes gobs of "guy juice" all over her spiky 'do, her chest, and just about everywhere else on the patio. There's definitely something hot about a guy unloading what looks like a year's worth of built-up sexual energy.

Satisfaction

It may seem paradoxical in a chapter on orgasms to discuss *not* having one. But, indeed, there are times when you may feel sexually satisfied without an orgasm. Occasionally, if the sex has been particularly intense, exhausting, or just plain exciting, the body may not have what you recognize as an orgasm, but feel satisfied anyway. Sometimes, your pleasure centers have had enough and they will let your body know it. And sometimes, especially if you have difficulty coming, you realize that it's not going to happen, so you just enjoy it for what it is and bask in the afterglow. If this should happen to you, then the Vivid Girls suggest a nap, a snack, or simply calling it a night. In no way should either partner take it as a sign of something else. Which brings us to the issue of faking it. Frankly, with your newfound freedom and all the tips picked up from this book, you shouldn't have to fake anything. And, women, be careful if you think guys can't tell the difference. Bobby says, "I like to see a woman get off when I'm eating her pussy. I can tell if a girl is faking or not. It's just a gut thing, really. But I don't think she's going to spend forty-five minutes with me eating her pussy if she isn't enjoying it. I like to lick their pussy and then that way, after I get off, I know she's been satisfied and can go to sleep." And don't forget that satisfaction doesn't always have to be accompanied by orgasm. Even supershooter Bobby doesn't always come. "Sometimes I've gotten them off but not come myself. I just say to them, 'No, I'm good.' It totally freaks them out and drives them crazy if I don't come. But, trust me, I had a good time."

Bobby brings up another tip that will earn guys bonus points: the guys in Vivid features always make sure the girl comes first. This little etiquette tip will help dispel any of those lingering stereotypes that guys just want to get themselves off first. It will also help ensure that the girl will do her very best to make sure the guy's orgasm is every bit as enjoyable as hers.

Afterward

After orgasm, some people (both male and female) like to roll over and go to sleep, while others like to smoke a cigarette, cuddle, or talk. "The payoff to a scene has always been the male orgasm," says Chi Chi. "That signifies the end of a scene. But in real life, there's no reason why you can't keep going with the foreplay for a little bit." But in the adult film world, he notes, "The afterglow is a towel and a shower." Kira says, "I like to fall asleep with his dick in my mouth; it's comforting." Jenna, on the other hand, prefers to nod out almost immediately. "I'm so much of a man because I'm one of those people who likes to roll over and go to sleep," she says. "You know how a lot of women like to cuddle and talk? For me, there's nothing left; I can't even form words. I'm not a big cuddler because I get so hot. I like to have my own space to think about what happened. I think men are the same way." Mercedez feels similarly to Jenna. "I'm the type who likes to go to sleep after it's done. I don't want to be held and talked to," she says. "I just want to go to bed." But she also notes she's occasionally energized afterward. "Sometimes my husband will hold me but I'm ready to get up and get out of bed. The perfect date for me would be a hotel; just walk in there, have sex, and then leave. That would be the perfect evening for me." Dasha adds, "I just like to lie there for a while, go slowly down, stare at the ceiling, and enjoy going down the wave. But my husband likes to go and wash himself, and then pat me and kiss me. If the guy likes to go to sleep, that's fine. I'll snuggle him. But if the guy would go to the couch and start watching TV, that would bum me out."

12
toys and trinkets

Fantasy File:

The cleaning lady returns to the custodian's office after emptying the trash from every office in the building. She nonchalantly plops a fancy shoe box she retrieved from a wastepaper basket down on the handsome young janitor's desk.

"How come I'm always the one working, and you're the one sitting on you ass?" she says.

The handsome janitor puts down the newspaper and opens the box. For a second, he is speechless; he can't believe his eyes. Inside the ordinary shoe box is a collection of all sorts of sex toys. He looks at the cleaning lady and wonders why such an exotic beauty is working as a cleaning lady. He can feel his dick beginning to harden.

"Are you freaking out on me again?" he asks gruffly, trying to mask his curiosity. His interest piqued, however, he begins to examine the items in the box and turns back toward her. "Disgusting," he exclaims.

"Hey," she playfully responds, "we might be able to use these."

She giggles a little, picks up the short red handle of what looks to be a horsehair whip, and dangles it in front of her, swinging it from side to side like a big, heavy cock.

"Hey, stop that," the janitor says, slightly sheepishly. Then he lifts something that looks like a coral mitten covered with rubber nibs out of the box. For a second, he imagines this is the same color as the inside of her pussy. He feels a little strange, but doesn't put it down.

Playfully, she extracts a small, vibrating egg out of the box and swings it in front of him. "Bend over, buddy," she says looking him straight in the eye, then laughs.

For a second, he stares at her, trying to decide if he should make a move. Then he realizes the rubber mitt is still on his hand. As she turns away from him, he reaches out and begins to slowly stroke her mahogany ass with the mitt.

She starts to object, but he sits her down on his lap gently and whispers, "Just relax."

Ever so slowly, he touches her breasts, then her nipples, with the nibs of the rubber mitt. It's a strange sensation at first, but it excites him nonetheless. She closes her eyes and leans her body back against his. He uses the mitt to explore further, reaching up under her thin cotton skirt, rubbing the mitt on her panties. She sighs. By this time he feels confident that she wants him, so he begins to lick her neck and ears, waiting to see what will happen.

The cleaning lady makes the next move. Standing and turning toward him, she strips off her clothes; then kneels to undo his fly and pull off his pants. She takes the head of his dick in her mouth and licks it from side to side, then puts her mouth over the corona and pops it in and out. From his vantage point sitting on the chair, he watches her head bob up and down, then grasps her hair and presses her face down on him. "Oh," he murmurs as she begins to rub the huge head of his cock with her nipple. He motions for her to sit on him, facing away. She lowers herself on his throbbing dick as he grasps her by the hips. Furiously, he pumps her up and down, up and down, on his cock. While in motion, he notices that she is looking at the two of them fucking in the large mirror hanging on the opposite wall. He watches her watching herself play with her petite breasts. He loves the sight of his cock going in and out of her.

With his dick still inside, he lifts her and carries over to his desk, laying her down so she is spread out before him. His thrusts become more urgent. She lifts her arms above her head and feels the box. Reaching inside, she pulls out the horsehair whip and hesitates for a moment. But at this point, he is too wild to object. He can only think about drilling his cock into her harder and harder. He grabs one of her ankles and puts it on his strong shoulder. She first begins dragging the horsehair over her breasts, then, as his hips start to buck, she begins to snap the whip harder over her body. He has never done anything like this before, but it makes him even harder and more excited. He rolls her over onto her stomach. Instinctively, she sits back on her haunches, rocks forward and steadies herself on all fours, and presents her dripping pussy to him. He enters her from behind, then grabs the handle out of her hand, and takes the pace up a notch. Faster, faster, using the whip as if he was a jockey riding a magnificent racehorse into the home stretch. Faster. He knows he can't last much longer. He pulls his wet cock out of her and pumps it several times with his hand, then shoots his creamy load on her ass.

★★ *from* The Audition,
directed by Ralph Parfait

The sex-toy industry has exploded over the past ten years as more couples search for ways to add some fun and variation to their love-making. The popularity of erotic accessories is reflected in adult movies, too, with vibrators, dildos, butt plugs, and other toys making regular appearances on-screen. Vivid even has its own comprehensive assortment, called Vivid Toys, that are made and distributed in adult bookstores by Doc Johnson. But some of the stars' favorites don't ever make it into a scene, especially vibrators that can obscure the close-up action of penetration, cover a performer's prettiest parts, or make too much noise. So, some toys are reserved for offscreen adventures, whether solo or with a lover. So here's a look at what you can shop for at your local adult toy retailer, or on the Internet, and what our experts have on their bedside tables.

> ❝ ❝ Toys just add more to a scene—they're fun, they are visually interesting, and, in my experience, women have great orgasms with them. ❞ ❞
>
> —*Chi Chi LaRue*

Chi Chi's right that sex toys enhance movie scenes, and they can add something to your private scenes as well. From an ordinary feather duster to a high-tech vibrator, erotic accessories add different sensations to the mix, spice up your sex routine, and can enhance orgasms for both partners. Tawny likes them for a change of pace. "Well, a toy is something different, something new to switch it up a bit," she says. "Plus, some guys really like to watch a girl get off with a sex toy." One of the nice things about toys is that you can use them all by yourself. Sunrise is a real sex toy enthusiast, and emphasizes the importance of using toys to masturbate: "I wake up in the morning and just think, hey, let's masturbate. Every female in America should have sex toys that suit her. You have to get those juices really working, or you will lose your ability to be in touch with your body, get wet, and have orgasms."

Remember, though, that toys are not just for those times when you're home alone; they can greatly enhance your sex life with your partner as well. Briana uses toys to spice up what she says is one of the most underrated sexual acts—mutual masturbation. "One of my favorite things in the world is to masturbate in front of my guy while he watches, then watch as he gets himself off. It really turns me on," she says. Toys can be used for mutual masturbation, manual stimulation, and all kinds of penetration, including vaginal and anal intercourse. Some toys are also perfectly suitable for use by either men or women.

> ❝ **Guys should be into playing with sex toys in bed. If a girl enjoys sex more, then he's having better sex, too.** ❞
>
> —Mercedez

Mercedez makes a valid point. Some guys might be intimidated by sex toys because they think bringing an erotic tool into the bedroom makes them seem inadequate, or they might feel like their own equipment isn't enough. Men, and women, should feel secure enough in themselves, the relationship, and their sexual skills that sex toys are a welcome addition, not something threatening. Briana agrees with Mercedez about the importance of embracing toys. "I couldn't date a man who was intimidated by sex toys," she says. "They spice up a relationship." If your man feels like toys will replace him or they are unnecessary, Savanna has this advice: "Make a guy feel secure and good about himself. If he's intimidated by a sex toy, let him know how much you want to use it and how great it's going to be. Plus, when you put a vibrator on your clit, he can feel it, too, so it's working for both of you."

If you're shy about introducing sex toys into the bedroom, you may want to ease into it with some simple things. For example, massage oil can add to an all-over body massage. Some oils are scented, others are flavored (some are both), so select a smell or a taste you and your partner like; plus many erotic oils warm up as you use them. Just remember not to use any kind of oil as a lubricant, since oils break down latex in condoms and can cause vaginal infections. And speaking of fragrance, Vivid Toys offers a variety of differently shaped and colored dildos, each with a matching scent of "joy jelly" such as guava pineapple, lemon lime, passion fruit, wild strawberry, and even mango orange.

Anything that creates different sensations against the skin, such as feathers, fur mitts, fingernails, and ice cubes, can add a sexy, unique dimension to foreplay. Novelties like erotic games, dirty dice, edible body paint, and underwear may seem silly, but they can actually jumpstart a sexy night, and fuel a new kind of exploration between you. And for sexy fun, Vivid even has Oral Blast Mint Oral Jel for "the ultimate blow job," and decks of naughty playing cards, guaranteed to heat up any game of bridge, hearts, and, of course, strip poker.

Vibrators

❝ My favorite vibrator is the pink Pocket Rocket. I like it, but it's too strong for me sometimes—also I have one that's silver and kind of thin, with a slight curve at the end, so that it just curves right around the clit. ❞

—Savanna

The most popular of all sensual tools, vibrators do exactly what their name suggests: they deliver consistent vibration, which relaxes muscles and stimulates genitals. Different vibrators create different sensations. Some are designed especially for women or men, while others can multitask. For many women, powerful, focused vibration on the pubic bone and clitoris, the clitoral hood, or on the clitoris itself is the best and fastest route to orgasm. A vibrator is an essential in anyone's bag of tricks, whether for use with a partner, or alone. Let's face it, there are just times when a woman feels sexy and there's no one around to play with.

Vibrators come in a wide variety of shapes and styles, from the sublime to the ridiculous. You might be surprised to know that some guys are intimidated by anything that looks even a tiny bit like a real penis—especially if he thinks it's larger than he is. These same guys, however, might be open to a vibrator that doesn't try to look like the real thing, such as a therapeutic-looking wand, a zebra-striped tube, a small finger cover, or something that looks like it came from *The Jetsons*. When one of the suburban dinner-party guests in the sex comedy *Nikki Loves Rocco* surprises a new houseguest by pulling a lime green vibrator with an attached clit stimulator out of the bathroom cabinet, the effect is upbeat, fun, and more than a little intriguing.

The shapes and styles of vibrators can be loosely organized into three categories based on what they do: external stimulators, penetrators, and multifunction vibrators. (Many of these types of Vivid Toys provide a combination of five functions: vibrate, roller-coaster, escalate, surge, and pulsate.) But there are other factors to consider when selecting a vibrator. These include: the way it looks (penis or bunny rabbit?); the power source (batteries vs. plug-in?); speed capabilities (one speed or many?); and noise level (hummer or lawn mower?). There's even a waterproof model you can take in the shower, one with a remote control, one that plugs into a USB computer port, and a Vivid "Glow in the Dark Pleasure Vibe"!

Vibrators designed especially for external clit stimulation come in two main types: portable and wand style. The portables are compact, battery-operated vibes that may be the size or shape of a large lipstick, a small egg, or a plastic dental flosser. One of the most popular examples, and a favorite of some of the Vivid crew, is the Pocket Rocket. Larger than a tube of mascara, but smaller than a Magic Marker, the Pocket Rocket (and toys with a similar design but different brand names) uses one battery and has one speed—on. Because it doesn't look like a giant penis, women who prefer discreet vibrators love this toy. If someone stumbled upon it in your house, they wouldn't think twice! Besides, Pocket Rockets are highly portable and can easily slip into a handbag or makeup case.

Similar to these are bullet- and egg-shaped vibes, like the Vivid Toys "Hot Shots," which are attached by a wire to a battery pack, which allows you to control the speed and, in some fancy varieties, the type of vibration. In recent years, there's been plenty of new, creative technology in the sex-toy industry. One new vibrator, for example, is activated solely by external sounds. In addition to the discretion factor, small vibrators can be great for use during intercourse because they don't get in the way of penetration. They have low to medium vibration speeds (in general, follow this rule: the more batteries, the more power), and many are very quiet. The downside for some women is that they may not pack enough punch.

Another portable variety of external stimulators is the vibrator designed to wear during intercourse. These toys—often aesthetically shaped like butterflies, ladybugs, or flowers—come with elastic straps that hold them in place, keeping the woman's vagina and ass free and clear for penetration. There are also small vibrators that slip over one or more of your fingers, turning someone's hand into a whole new stimulating machine in its own right.

Wand-style vibrators, often sold in stores as neck massagers, are bigger and more powerful than their portable sisters. The most popular brand of this type is the Hitachi Magic Wand, but Panasonic makes something similar called the Panabrator, and there's also an industrial-strength model with double heads. Wand vibrators usually have large rounded heads with plenty of surface area to cover the clitoris and surrounding area. Electric, like the Hitachi, or rechargeable wand vibrators don't mess around—they deliver very strong concentrated vibrations in variable intensities. Some women swear they can't live (or come) without them, while others find them imposing and way too powerful. Because of their size, they work well with manual stimulation à deux or solo, but take some creative positioning to use with a partner (try doggie style or spooning). The downside to the wands is lack of portability, or getting tangled up in the electrical cord.

Phallic-shaped vibrators are built for penetration, and curved phallic vibes are ideal for G-spot stimulation. In addition to variable speeds, the one thing these have in common is their shape: hard plastic versions looks like oversize lipstick tops and can be metallic, leopard-printed, or candy-colored. Flexible rubber or silicone ones may be designed to resemble penises, or they can take the form of just about anything, from a dolphin to a chili pepper. There are also phallic-shaped vibrators made of hard plastic that come with a re-movable, soft rubber sleeve. Tawny prefers this type of toy: "I know a lot of girls use vibrators on their clits, but I really like them for pene-tration, especially the curved toys. Because of their shape, they hit my G-spot perfectly." And if you're not exactly sure whether you prefer a vibrator for vaginal, anal, or G-spot stimulation, there's a Vivid Toy combo pack that includes a multispeed vibrator along with a vaginal sleeve, an anal sleeve, a G-spot sleeve, and a bottle of Vivid Girls "Lube of Choice." Phallic vibes, especially the firm kind, can also be used for clitoral stimulation, but more often they produce less powerful vibra-tions. Moreover, if the really cheap ones are used with too much force or pressure, they can break apart at just the wrong moment. Briana says she likes to use two vibrators at once for maximum pleasure. "I like to use the Pocket Rocket and a slim, firm dildo together," she notes. "The Pocket Rocket goes on my clit, and the tip of the vibra-tor in my butt, and I am in ecstasy."

❝ ❝ I love the Jack Rabbit vibe—it hits two spots at the same time. ❞ ❞

—Kira

Dual-action vibrators combine both styles in one toy. They are phallic for penetration, and they have an attachment for external stim-ulation as well. This dildo-vibrator combination, with such names as Rabbit Pearl, Jack Rabbit, or Techno Rabbit, is universally praised by all the Vivid Girls, and several of these are available from Vivid Toys. The reason they are best known as "rabbits" is because the most pop-ular type of dual-action vibrator has a rotating shaft filled with plastic pearls (imagine a gumball machine) and a small rabbit whose ears vi-brate against the clit when the toy is inserted in the pussy. It's one of Savanna's favorites for quickies: "I do have this beautiful white vibra-tor that I use by myself, only if I don't have a lot of time. It has pearls that go around inside it and a clit stimulator—so you put the shaft in and then get your clit stimulated also."

★VIVID GIRL★ FAVORITES:

VIBRATORS WE LOVE

Briana: "The Pocket Rocket is my favorite. If girls haven't tried it, they absolutely should—it's the best."

Dasha: "I filmed a movie with a rabbit vibrator and I liked it so much, I took it home with me!"

Jenna: "Pocket-size vibes are good for taking with you when you travel, so you're not embarrassed if they search your luggage!"

Sunrise: "The rabbit hits all my sensitive spots—my G-spot, my clit—at the same time."

Kira: "The little vibrating eggs—I always liked those. I use them both with a partner and by myself."

Tawny: "I've got a slim, curvy G-spot vibrator that sends my body into overdrive!"

Jenna loves her dual-action vibe so much, she has to keep replacing it. "I have so many vibrators because I get a lot of toys for free, so I've tested them all!" she says. "But my good old trusty Techno Rabbit always comes through. It has the dildo that rotates and a vibrator that works your clit, so it does everything at once. A person can't do it as well or for as long. I've broken at least fifty Techno Rabbits. My partner always knows when it's broken because the batteries have mysteriously been taken out of all the remote controls in the house. Always keep a healthy supply of batteries!" Savanna warns women to use vibrators in moderation: "I recommend that women have an on-again, off-again relationship with their vibrator so they don't get too dependent."

Often, when a woman uses a vibrator to stimulate her clitoris during intercourse, a man can feel the waves of vibrations as he penetrates her, adding yet another dimension to his pleasure. Plus, you can use portable and wand-style external vibrators to stimulate his balls, the shaft of the penis, or the head. Just be aware that most guys prefer the vibes set on low. And, because guys shouldn't feel left out, there are vibrating toys designed especially for men, including vibrating penis pumps, vibrating sleeves that engulf and stimulate the penis, and cup-shaped vibrators designed to stimulate the sensitive head of the penis. There are even vibes that work on both of you at the same time: vibrating cock rings are made of plastic, rubber, or jelly rubber. They slide over the shaft of the penis, and have a bullet-shaped vibrator or textured nub on top that vibrates the dick and buzzes the clit during intercourse. Sex-toy manufacturers are always improving technology and selection to ensure there's a vibrator for everyone; they are waterproof, remote-controlled, designer, and even crafted to look like your favorite fountain pen, so find one with the features that are just right for you.

Dildos

Dildos are phallic toys for penetration, and like vibrators, they come in all shapes and sizes. There are dildos that strive to look as realistic as possible, with veins, balls, and circumcised heads, and there are ones that look nothing like a penis—sparkled, striped, or swirled with bright colors. There are straight ones, curved ones, long ones, fat ones, and even S-curved ones designed to tickle a woman's G-spot. They also come in a variety of materials, including plastic, rubber, glass, and Plexiglas. Some are even interchangeable and designed to fit into a harness.

Many women like to use dildos during masturbation. They are also good tools for foreplay, as a slim dildo can help her get aroused, and get her pussy or ass ready for your cock. Mercedez loves her dildo collection for the variety it brings to her sex life: "The thing I love about dildos is that you can try out all different sizes without going out and sleeping with other men. Dildos give me options." Speaking of options, dildos are also a great way to experiment with double penetration without having to invite another person into the mix. And if you would like to double your pleasure, there are always toys like Vivid's Double Dong, which, they say, you can "use alone, or get connected and share the fun."

In the suspenseful drama *Swoosh,* you can see two different types of dildos. The one that shows up poolside is a strap-on, which we'll get to a little later on. The other, a blue gel dildo, is used by a man in another scene to get a woman excited before fucking her. In *Where the Boys Aren't 14* and *Where the Boys Aren't 15,* lots of toys are used. In these two all-girl films, you'll see both hard (plastic or metal) and soft (rubber or gel) models, used in a variety of activities and combinations. For example, there's one girl inserting a dildo in and out of another girl, there's dildo sucking (sometimes a sexy turn on), a double-ended double-duty model enjoyed by two girls at once, as well as a variety of anal toys. What's amazing and fun to see is the seemingly endless variety of shapes, colors, sizes, and models all used in a single film.

Love Beads and Other Anal Toys

Although they don't come in as many varieties as vibrators and dildos, there are still plenty of anal toys to choose from. A butt plug can either be something that's inserted in the rectum and stays there throughout the sex act to give that person a feeling of being "full," or it can be something that, after insertion, is manipulated in and out like a dildo. There are also battery-pack models that twirl around and tickle your insides. Most anal toys have a basic shape that looks like a slender Christmas tree; narrow at the top, gently widening, then, toward the bottom, back in again and out again, sort of like a tree trunk and root-ball. The reason for this is that they can go in as far as one wants. The "trunk" and "root-ball" parts, akin to a neck and shoulders, provide something to hold on to, and prevent it from getting lost up there. Vivid Toys specifically designed to stimulate this region include an anal screw, a smooth anal tool, a vibrating and waterproof smooth anal toy, and a six-inch anal starter.

Love beads are made up from a series of small balls strung together and spaced about one to three inches apart. They may strike us as new, but this idea has actually been around for a very long time, having originated in ancient Japan, where pearls were the "ball" of choice. Love beads are basically an anal toy that can be used by both men and women. You lube them up, insert them in the rectum, and pull them out one at a time at appropriate moments. Vivid's versions come in three different colors and sizes of balls (S, M, L), and have a ring at one end to hold on to for easy extraction. Love beads should not be confused with something that is sort of a cross between a dildo and love beads, a orbed butt plug, which is basically either a flexible or rigid dildo shaped like several marbles glued together in a row. This also comes in a descending orb model, so the small balls go in first, and as the anus relaxes, larger ones can be inserted. They are also designed this way so they can't get lost up there. You can view many of these type of toys in the voyeuristic film *Looking In,* and also in *Where the Boys Aren't 14* and *Where the Boys Aren't 15.* To experience a variety of anal sensations with toys, however, you might want to check out one of Vivid's multispeed "Anal Adventure" kits, which contain a six-inch pearl purple vibrator, jelly anal beads, a jelly anal plug, a slim butt plug, long and short vibrator sleeves, and special lube.

Strap-ons

Strap-ons are dildos that fit into a harness that is strapped around a woman's pelvis. Their allure is that a woman can play around with being the "fucker" instead of always being the "fuckee." They are usually used, both in adult movies and real life, for girl-on-girl action. However, there are some heterosexual guys who, from time to time, like the tables turned. A woman using a strap-on with a guy certainly goes farther than inserting her finger in his rectum, but there are definitely some men who want to experience the full sensation. And as Chi Chi says, it's not gay and doesn't look gay if a woman is doing it.

You can see a strap-on being worn and used in *Looking In* during one of the group sex scenes. But one of the sexiest images is Briana wearing one in *Swoosh.* At the beginning of the film, Briana takes part in a large of poolside orgy, gets thirsty, and goes inside the house only to find there's no more orange juice. There is definitely something exotic about "chicks with dicks," but Briana looks especially adorable checking out the refrigerator with the strap-on bouncing up and down under her skirt. Later in the movie, Briana is arrested (still wearing it) and taken to the jailhouse. In the script, this prompts a series of dream sequences in which the strap-on is quite prominent.

One of the cutest Vivid Toys offered is the Ultra Harness, with a six-inch pink crystal jelly dong and an adorable pink leather harness. And one of the most unique strap-ons is Vivid's Blue Jelly Devil Tongue, which touts "equal pleasure where you need it most."

Clips and Piercings

Many men and women enjoy a really tight and consistent pinch to their nipples during sex, and sometimes their partners just don't have enough hands to do everything. Nipple clips and vibrating nipple teasers can be the answer. These are often attached before sex, and can be yanked off in one fell swoop by a cord that connects them. The better models allow you to adjust the tightness of the clips. In the same vein, clit clips, which look something like an elongated bobby pin, do the same thing.

Nipple, navel, labia, clit, penis, and tongue piercings don't technically qualify as merely toys, but they do affect sex by affording somewhat different sensations for both the giver and the recipient. Those who have them say that piercings heighten feeling in, and awareness of, that specific area of their body. And recipients of oral sex from someone with a pierced tongue say the sensation of a cold, hard, metal bead feels great combined with that of a smooth, hot tongue.

❝ ❝ I had my nipples pierced and I love to watch someone sucking on my nipples. ❞ ❞

—Savanna

Savanna has a tongue piercing that you can see her use in *Good Time Girl*. The writer who is the leading male character in *Obsession* uses his pierced tongue for some slurping oral action, too. And the newest customer at the all-girl garage in *Where the Boys Aren't 15* uses her pierced tongue to "rim" the pretty mechanic's butt.

Other Toys

We already mentioned G-spot stimulators and butt plugs in this chapter, and the variety of cock rings in another chapter, but there are still more toys to explore. With most of these items, just the idea of using them can be as arousing as the sensations they create.

Ben Wa balls are an old, Japanese, low tech version of internal vibrators. Each ball (there are usually two or three) contains a weight that allows it to "roll around." Ben Wa balls are inserted into the vagina and can be worn all day, any day, and for whatever length of time, without anyone knowing they're there.

Simple blindfolds are an old favorite based on the idea that sex is more exciting if you don't know what's coming next, and also, that without sight, all of a person's senses are focused on touch. Other old favorites are wrist cuffs and ankle cuffs, which offer the same effect as metal handcuffs, but are a lot gentler to wear. The idea of these is that one person is in control, and the other is somewhat helpless.

And last, there are the toys

TOY TIPS

One word of caution: silicone lubricants are incompatible with silicone sex toys; the lube and toy will bond to each other, and the toy will be permanently ruined, so stick to water-based lubes only, or, if you want to use silicone lube, cover your silicone toys with a latex condom.

1. Always use lube with vibrators, dildos, and butt plugs.
2. Silicone toys are the easiest to disinfect.
3. Store toys in a clean, cool, dry place.
4. Clean rubber and gel toys after each use with warm water and antibacterial soap.
5. Rubber is porous. It can be cleaned, but not completely disinfected.
6. Never share your toys with others unless you slip a condom on them first.
7. Silicone is not porous. Clean and disinfect toys with hot water and antibacterial soap; or boil them for three minutes; or put them in the top rack of the dishwasher.
8. Thermal plastic (better known by brand names like CyberSkin and UltraSkin) is porous. Keep it free of bacteria by using a condom each time, or don't share it.

that begin to veer a little into S&M or B&D (sadism, masochism, bondage and discipline). We're not talking about superserious equipment here; just stuff for power fantasies and role-playing. At Vivid, none of the movies ever get into anything that's really rough, degrading, or humiliating to either men or women. A small, flat paddle is a favorite for some "naughty schoolboy" or "stern headmistress" play, or as an alternative to a flat palm for light spanking. Similarly, a soft, short handled latex whip (which actually looks more like a cheerleading pom-pom) can be used to put a blush on one's partner's nether parts if used lightly, or it can leave marks if used with more force. A Vivid movie that has scenes with a similar whip is *Blondage,* but it's obvious that the whip is being used as part of a stage act. If you think you'd like to try out this type of role-playing, Vivid Toys offers something called a Bondage and Slave Kit that contains everything you need: a small whip with a handle, a slave leash, wrist and ankle restraints, a collar, and a bridle gag. And speaking of Kits, Vivid also has Overnighter Kits, Adventure Kits, Dare Essentials Kits, and even an Ultimate Masturbation Kit.

> ❝ I have a house full of sex toys. They are a big part of my sexuality, and I love them. ❞
>
> —*Sunrise*

13
mixing it up

Fantasy File:

Tired but restless after moving into their new home all day, he goes downstairs and steps outside for some fresh air. Standing in front of the house, he looks around the quiet neighborhood. He feels something in the air that excites him, and he instinctively glides his hand over his cock, which slowly awakens under his boxer briefs. Then, feeling self-conscious, he looks up and down the street to make sure no one has seen him.

Across the way, he sees one of his new neighbors through the window: a dark-haired woman in a short red robe. She stands facing the window, then opens up her robe to reveal her huge, cushiony breasts. For a moment, he thinks he should turn away, but there's something in the woman's stance that leads him to believe she wants to be watched. He continues to stare at her. She massages her breasts and neck, then reaches down under her robe, where she lightly tickles her pussy. She turns around, hikes up her robe, and bends forward, revealing for him the voluptuous mounds of her ass. He glances over to his left, and sees his next-door neighbors also watching the mysterious woman in red. Completely unself-conscious, they wave hello to one another. Embarrassed, he runs back inside his house. But he can't/doesn't want to stop looking, so he goes into the living room and continues to watch her through his window.

He hears his wife coming down the stairs. As she walks into the room, she looks only at him. Feeling slightly guilty about his watching, he turns her back to the window and kisses her, even though he can't resist watching his provocative neighbor over his wife's shoulder. "Kiss me," he says, and she does. She feels his erection as she leans into him. They kiss again. He looks back across the street. The neighbor, deprived of an audience, ties up her robe and walks away.

His wife, meanwhile, massages his cock through his shorts, then kneels down in front of him. She breathes warmly on the swelling package inside, then pulls his dick out through the fly. She takes him into her mouth and massages his shaft at the same time. He places his hands on her shoulders, and begins thrusting into her warm, sensuous mouth. For a second, he wonders whether anyone is watching him. To his surprise, the thought excites him and he feels his cock grow even bigger and harder as his wife continues to suck on it. Maybe the move to a new neighborhood will be good for their marriage, after all, he thinks as she lovingly glides his dick in and out of her mouth.

★★ *from* Looking In,
directed by Paul Thomas

For those who watch porn, as for those who like to watch any movie, there is always an element of fantasy. Whether we are buying into the fantasy plot, or simply want to see some hot bodies engaged in hot action, there is an undeniable excitement that comes just from watching. The scenarios portrayed in movies may inspire you to enact your own erotic drama. Beyond the sexual techniques and positions we mentioned before, there are some other elements—some physical, some more psychological—that you can incorporate into your own life.

Roughing It

Rough sex can mean a lot of different things to different people. It can range from a playful erotic wrestling match to the subtle domination of hair pulling and the occasional smack on the ass. Regardless of what it means to you, it's necessary for both partners to be into it. Try to gauge your partner's mood. Have you been very physical with each other before? What are our expectations for the evening? If your partner is looking forward to a romantic dinner followed by a soothing soak in a hot tub, then a bout of erotic wrestling might be the last thing they want to do. But if the mood is right and the energy level is high, then a bit of roughhousing can be fun and exhilarating. As an aside, we want to make clear that what we are discussing here is not meant to be violent or harmful, but playful and adventurous, and that Vivid movies do not feature violence.

"Rough" in this case means things like hair tugging, biting, and spanking. If you want to get into some rougher stuff, you need to let your partner know. If you want something done a little harder or more forcefully, say so. In the heat of the moment, lines like "fuck me harder" don't sound silly at all; to a lot of people they sound totally hot. Sometimes you can communicate what you want without words. "I have this look that I tend to give that people say they can tell when I want it harder. I've had two partners tell me that there's one look that I pass off when I want it mild and one for when I want it rough that says, 'Why aren't you pounding me?'" says Kira.

Let's say you want to raise the intensity of your kissing. If you are behind your partner, try biting them on the back of the neck and shoulder. A tip: don't bite too hard; use only your front teeth; hold the bite just for a second and then let go. If your partner responds favorably, go a little bit harder. Some people love the sensation of being bitten during sex, and some love it only during a particular kind of lovemaking. "Every once in a while I like it rough. I really like hard biting on my back and neck, almost like bruises. It just really gets me going," Dasha explains. Other places to sink your teeth into include the nipples, the buttocks, and the inner thighs. In all these areas, the idea is to start softly and then go a little harder. You may end up going even further than you thought. As Chi Chi puts it, "I love nipple biting. You sink your teeth in it and pull it out as far as it can go."

The next way to mix things up is hair pulling, which can be a big turn-on for some men and women. Sometimes just a tight grip during a vigorous massage will do the trick. Or, start while you are kissing, slide your hand into your partner's hair, and tighten your grip. If they melt into your arms, then you know it's working. Briana enjoys the rough-and-ready school. "I love rough sex. Grab me, shove me against the wall, and just have your way with me. I get so turned on. I like it when a guy just tears my clothes off; I like having my hair pulled. It keeps things exciting," she says.

Briana brings up another point. Sometimes, it's not a specific bite, tug, or pull, but just a general "manhandling" of your partner, only the handler can be a man or a woman. Lots of people like the concept of being "thrown up against the wall" and it's a staple of film fantasies. Hard kissing, tight squeezing, extra-vigorous massaging, holding your partner's hands so they can't move them—all of these are things you might normally do, just not as forcefully. "I like guys who are forceful in bed. Not forceful to the point where I'm like 'what are you doing?'—just strong and vigorous," says Mercedez, adding, "If I'm doggie style, I like him to grab my shoulders." Tawny and Dasha express similar enthusiasm. "Throw me on the bed, pull my hair, take control of the scene and me. I like the feeling that someone is taking advantage of me," says Tawny. Dasha also likes a guy to "throw me on the bed and take me" every once in a while.

Speaking of doggie style, if you're back there, you'll have a great view of your partner's ass. Ever considered spanking it a little? As always, start lightly and then go a little harder if your partner seems to like it. For many people, a spank when they are very aroused adds to their excitement. "I'm into spanking as long as it's during sex," says Kira. Tawny likes it, too. "I love to be spanked," she says. "For me it's part of submitting to my partner and of them having their way with me." In *Blondage,* during their stage show, the two girls engage in a lot of rough play; they push each other around, pull each other's hair, and deliver quite a few spanks to the ass. And in *The Vision,* the sexy girls from the past—Cleopatra, Helen of Troy, and, especially, bossy bitch Delilah—get their share of fanny whacks. As we discussed in Chapter

9, love taps should be delivered with your whole hand open. Aim right for the middle of the cheek, where you'll get a resounding slap noise when you make contact.

For other areas, you need to be a bit more cautious. Chi Chi says, "I love a little pussy or asshole spanking—just a little slap on the genitals is hot to me." For this move, you can't use your whole hand, so use the flat part of your fingers. Since the parts are extra sensitive and will be even more so during sex, the delivery here is more of tap than a slap. You can see the lawyer do it to one of the three daughters in *Filthy Rich*. In addition to tapping and slapping is snapping. Chi Chi loves to film "a thing I call snapping. If the guy is superhard, the hottest thing for me is when a girl grabs hold of it hard, pulls it down, and lets it snap back up to hit him in the stomach. It's rough yet it's so hot because you see how hard the guy is."

"Grab my arms, pull them behind my back, push my head down on the bed. Rough sex is good for me as long as it's not too rough. I like a guy to take control, but know that I am really the one in control," says Kira. One note of caution for rough players: for partners with any history or abuse, rough stuff in bed can be totally off-limits. So be respectful of their needs. You want whatever you do to be playful and sexy, not harmful. Kira's point is well taken for making rough play consensual and fun: you create the illusion of giving up control, but know that you can stop it at any time.

You're on a Role

❝ To make the fantasies have enough fuel to them to be exciting, once in a while you need to make them real. ❞

—Paul Thomas, Vivid director

Fantasy role-playing is not only a way to add variety to your lovemaking, but also a tool to explore a different "character" within yourself, a new dynamic between you and your partner, or a wild setup completely different from your normal life. For some people, the images and scenarios they picture in their heads, or watch on the screen during masturbation, will always remain in the realm of fantasy. Others need only take a small step to turn a fantasy into reality. Indeed, with porn becoming increasingly common, a lot of people are doing things every day that were once considered the special province of the porn star.

Kira encourages people to have open minds about fantasies and role-playing. "I didn't realize how many fantasies and fetishes are out there. I know what it's like to be the conservative girl, uncomfortable trying new things. Since I've been in the business, I am more accepting. Everyone has their own likes and dislikes. Some things I might be willing to try; others, I know I'm not into. But I wouldn't judge someone else for it," she explains.

The first step to putting your role-playing fantasy into production is to talk it over with your partner. You can't coerce them into trying something they don't want to do, so you need to listen to what they *do* want to do. Paul suggests talking about it in detail beforehand. "If you're really going out on the edge, a written agreement might not be a bad idea. Two people have to know what the parameters are; they need to acknowledge they're playing with fire. Events may happen that weren't talked about beforehand," he cautions.

Once you've agreed that you both want to take the next step, fantasy role-playing is a fun way to bring erotic ideas to life. Even though trying on different roles gives you the chance to be someone else for the evening, it can ultimately bring you closer together. As you work to maintain the scenario, you cooperate and build something together. To play out your fantasies, all you need is imagination, communication, and a sense of playfulness.

The majority of role-playing fantasies involve some kind of power game. Think of some of the most popular ones: doctor and patient, teacher and student, millionaire and maid, housewife and pool boy. They all center on one of the figures having some sort of power over the other. Think about some of the scenarios—from books, movies, or your own mind—that have turned you on in the past. Have you daydreamed of having a lover worship you as an erotic servant would? Did you always want to be the quarterback who gets the head cheerleader? Do you imagine picking up a total stranger in a bar and taking him home? Mercedez likes to take her job of exotic dancer to another level at home. "I dress up in my dance clothes and leave my heels on. I give him a 'table dance' and it turns into sex," she admits. Other people get aroused by the idea of doing something naughty or taboo, like spanking or bondage. "You have to find somebody you trust," notes Bobby, adding that rough sex is not abuse. Instead, he says, "All the rough stuff is about sending you to that place together. It's got a kind of ritual to it and it's all about the forbidden." The sex-with-a-stranger fantasy is one many couples act out. They go to a bar separately, flirt with each other, and then go home together as if meeting for the first time. Mercedez indulges in this fantasy with her partner from time to time. "The actual first time we had sex, I had to take over. He was scared and nervous. I had to grab him and show him what I liked. We were exploring each other's body for the first time, and it was really hot." Now they fantasy-flirt in public and go home together as a way of reenacting that initial encounter.

The fun of many roles is that you can play with power in a way that you can't in real life. Perhaps you fantasize about surrendering to another person, being taken against your will, or being forced to do something. "I like when people do things to me, undress me, have their way with me," explains Tawny. Sunrise gets off on the idea of someone taking her by surprise. "It really turns me on to pretend that I'm asleep, and my guy just starts messing with me," she confesses.

Maybe you want to be in control, calling the shots, and have your partner worship you. Bobby says he is usually the dominant one in a fantasy, but "if a woman wanted to do something crazy like that to me, that would be fine. The important thing is to have trust and passion." Bobby gets to act out just such a scene in the film-within-the-film in *Good Things*. Dominatrix Briana bosses him around, slaps him up and

VIVID GIRL FAVORITES:

down, and uses him like a sex toy. Whether in character or just as an occasional add-on during your normal sex sessions, ordering your partner to do something, especially something they don't normally do, can be really exciting.

Just remember that what happens in the bedroom stays in the bedroom. In other words, it's not about one partner actually being dominant or submissive, but about *playing* these roles. Dasha likes to play both roles. "I like to be wild, throw a man on the bed, leap on him, hold his hands down, and do it. I like playing different roles. I also like it when a guy is like that and makes me feel totally helpless. Just throw me on the bed and take me."

Show-and-Tell

Voyeurism and exhibitionism are two other areas that can help mix things up. In our visually saturated world, many of us have become accidental voyeurs. We are so used to seeing hot, barely clothed models on every billboard, magazine cover, and TV show that it barely registers as sexy. But the fact is, we like to watch. If we didn't, then porn wouldn't be a multibillion-dollar industry. Quite a few porno flicks actually play on our compulsion to watch others. *So I Married a Porn Star* is a humorous look at men's obsession with porn. The main character meets his porn-star wife while she's stripping at a bar. She keeps her other work a secret, but the guy finds out when his buddies see her in a video they pop in while playing poker. *Blondage* takes place in a strip club, and the main sex scene involves the two hot blondes putting on a show for the randy male customers. Another scene features two male bar patrons who end up doing it onstage with the stripper.

Looking In is all about voyeurism. The new neighbor can't resist checking out the hot chick in the window across the way, but it ends up helping him get it on with his wife, with whom he's having bedroom problems. Conversely, later in the film, it comes out that the couple he watches are exhibitionists, and that they like to get off with other people watching. In our culture of proudly buffed bodies, you're likely to encounter a few people with exhibitionist tendencies yourself. This can range from a bold public display of affection on the beach to posting home sex videos on the Internet.

If you want to test the waters of voyeurism at home, try watching your partner masturbate. If you're the masturbator, you need to pretend that you are alone. Don't stare at your partner and don't be self-conscious. Just do whatever you would normally do, and maybe your partner will even pick up a tip or two. Some couples experiment with this by watching each other through a keyhole or from the closet. If you're the watcher, it's okay to stroke yourself as you watch, but keep quiet if you want to maintain the illusion that your partner is unaware of your presence. Many people fantasize about seeing their partner with someone else. Paul admits: "I am obsessed with seeing the woman that I care for with another man." If you're not ready to watch your partner with someone else, then maybe you can do some watching together, and a Vivid video is a good place to start.

If you want to get in touch with your exhibitionist side, you might want to check out a sex party. It need not be as kinky and leathery as the one in *Obsession;* in fact, quite a few happen in regular old suburban homes. You don't have to swap if you don't want to, but you and your partner can have an audience and an orgasm at the same time. Others like to be seen, but don't want to know who's watching. The perfect setup for them would be an apartment in a Manhattan high-rise, where hundreds of neighbors you'll never meet can see right into your window. Do it near the window, and surely you'll find a voyeur or two who will want to watch.

14
pushing the envelope

Fantasy File:

It's another typical Saturday night in the suburbs. Four couples get together at Joe and Cathy's house for the usual dinner party, and already, Al's wife, Anne, has made some catty remarks about the crudités.

Joe takes Al aside and says, "You've got to help me. Can't we do something about these boring parties? The wives all try to outdo each other in the kitchen. We have some hors d'oeuvres; we stuff ourselves, we get drunk, and we go home, and what? We feel miserable the next morning. Let's do something different, something exciting for a change. This is boring."

Al, looking a little nerdy in his polo shirt, glasses, and chinos, thinks about what Joe has just said. Letting his mind run free for a second, he fantasizes that his neighbor Chuck is buck naked with a huge boner, being led around like a dog on a leash.

"What are you two guys talking about?" interrupts Anne.

"Nothing, honey," replies Al, snapping back to reality.

Ding-dong. The two people standing outside the front door are very eager because, after driving for some time, they believe they have finally found the right house for what is to be their first swingers party. Cathy, wearing a dowdy white dress, answers the door and welcomes them.

"Hi, I'm Tom Johnson and this is my wife, Cindy," he says, grabbing Cathy and giving her a little cuddle. "Wow, you're hot," he adds. Cathy is a little taken aback, but aiming to be the quintessential hostess, she welcomes them inside.

After introductions are made, Cindy, a blond bombshell in a leopard-print shirt, black bra, and thigh-high patent-leather boots, strokes Chuck's face. "You're cute," she murmurs seductively. "We're going to have fun tonight."

"Who are they?" asks Anne.

"I have no idea," Cathy replies.

"Well, aren't you worried?"

Cathy thinks for a moment. "Well, maybe they're the people who moved into the McIntyre house?"

"No," says Anne, "I've already met them."

"Well, I can't just kick them out," says Cathy as she moves to the living room to join her guests.

Cindy rummages through her bag. "I brought some vegetables," she says, handing Cathy a phallic-shaped cucumber and a banana. "Oh, and something else, too."

Cathy reads the name on the video Cindy hands her as a hostess gift: "*Hot Asses #6*, hmmm."

"I hope you don't have that one already," says Tom. "It's our favorite."

The suburban guys begin to fantasize about the possibilities. Al conjures up an image of sexy Cindy stroking him as his wife looks on. Meanwhile, Joe thinks about what he'd like to do with Chuck's wife. He imagines her bent over the powder-room sink with a tiny lace thong that he pushes aside to lick her ass and pussy. "Oh, yeah, lap it up," he imagines her saying to him. Then he fantasizes how he would order her to lick her fingers and rub her own pussy. "How would you like me to stick my tongue in your ass?" he thinks. "Yeah, rub that little butt hole. You like it when I stick my tongue in your ass, huh?" He daydreams of receiving a long, sweet blow job right before he fucks the living daylights out of her. His reverie of their steamy lovemaking is broken as Tom appears snapping a photo of the two in action.

"That was quite a performance," Tom says admiringly. "You're an incredible fuckster, and I'm an amateur. But it's nice to have someone to look up to. I just hope I can be as effective tonight." As fantasy blends with reality, and not knowing exactly what to make of all this, Joe continues to concentrate on the head bobbing up and down on his cock. "Oh, fuck," he cries as he shoots his load.

Meanwhile, back in the dining room, Cathy serves the main course.

"How long have you guys been fucking each other?" asks Tom matter-of-factly.

"What did you say?" says Joe as the other diners look askance at one another.

Tom thinks for a second. "Let me rephrase that. How long have you guys been having sex with each other?"

By this time, the champagne and wine have broken down some neighborly inhibitions, and everyone laughs off the remark.

Tom, in all earnestness, turns to Anne and says, "You're really beautiful. I can't wait to have sex with you." Then, turning respectfully toward Al, he says, "You don't mind if I fuck your wife, Al?"

Meanwhile, Cindy sashays over to the other side of the table and says to Chuck, "I can tell you're the wild man," as she nuzzles his face between her breasts. "Now why don't you show me just how wild you are?"

"I think there's a little miscommunication here," says Al, jumping into the conversation for a last-ditch attempt at normality.

"I can take care of myself," his wife replies, enjoying the attention from her newfound admirer.

As Cathy asks about whether there are too many spices in the casserole, Cindy ignores them. She shows her unbridled enthusiasm for swinging as she sucks Chuck's thick cock with vigor and delight.

Trying to ignore Cindy down on the floor between Chuck's legs, Cathy asks the others, "So, what do you guys want to do?" Meanwhile, still seated in his dinner chair, Chuck lifts Cindy up and down and slams his dick into her.

"Watch," is the unanimous answer.

Chuck lifts Cindy and switches positions so she is in his chair, her black boots and thighs spread out wide as he buries his shaft deep inside her. By this time, Tom has made his move toward Chuck's wife, who obliges him by taking the head of his cock into her mouth. Not to be left out, Joe begins to play with Cathy's clit and she leans back and moans with pleasure. By this time, Cindy's head and shoulders pound on the floor as her ass lifts higher and higher to meet Chuck's urgent thrusts. The finale begins when Chuck comes on her voluminous breast mounds.

"Well, Chuck," says Al, "I guess you give new meaning to 'after-dinner entertainment.' "

One Year Later

Brad and Audrey, an attractive young couple who have recently relocated to the community, make their way to their car as they prepare to go out for the evening.

"So what do you think they'll be like?" asks Audrey.

"Oh, probably some stuffy fuddy-duddies," answers Brad. "We'll be playing canasta by the end of the evening and I'm sure we'll be the wildest ones there."

Meanwhile, back at Cathy and Joe's house, Cathy and Cindy put on a sexy little striptease for Joe and Al, pressing their asses and breasts into a glass wall partition. Cathy, wearing nothing but a red crinoline and a black bustier, and Cindy, in a white micro-miniskirt, cavort unself-consciously with each other. Cindy sits on the floor while Cathy stands above her, spreading her legs so Cindy can lick her snatch and ass. Cindy wraps one arm around Cathy's leg. She puts her index fingers together and, with one deft motion, rubs them back and forth like a washcloth on Cathy's slit. Never a party pooper, Tom goes to join them as Joe, Al, and Anne watch the show.

"Boy, things have really changed in the past year," comments Joe.

Anne, dressed in a gauzy mesh dress with nothing underneath except her black bikini panties, massages Al's growing hard-on. "Yeah," replies Al, "I went from Dockers to leather."

They watch as Tom skillfully undresses both women, holding Cindy's leg up against the wall while Cathy voraciously devours his dick.

"It's really exciting to watch a forty-two-year old guy making it with two young girls," says Joe as Al and Anne nod in agreement.

"Hey, did you fuck my wife yet?" asks Al.

"Sure, don't you remember the four of us in this room last year?" answers Joe.

Next Cindy sucks Cathy's pussy as Cathy sucks Tom's big cock dry. Cathy plays with Cindy's clit as Cindy licks her husband's huge balls. They change positions so Tom can fuck Cindy better while Cathy tweaks Cindy's nipples and licks her neck and breasts.

The doorbell rings just as Tom shoots his wad all over Cindy and Cathy.

"Who's that?" someone asks.

"Oh, I forgot, the new people, the Thorsens," says

Cathy, smoothing her hair and skirt. "I met her at the super-
market, and ran into them at the library yesterday. They
seems like a nice enough couple—and they're both cute."

"Hi, come in," says Joe, opening the door for Brad
and Audrey, and introducing them around.

"Audrey," asks Tom, "have you ever had a man lick
champagne from your tits?"

★★ *from* Nikki Loves Rocco,
directed by Paul Thomas

Threesomes and Groups

❝❝ Something I did for the first time
on camera and now can't live without
is having sex with two people at once.
I fantasized about it a lot beforehand.
When it actually happened, it was so
great! I love to be the center of
attention and ravished! ❞❞

—*Savanna*

If you've watched many adult movies, you know that there is usually
at least one scene that involves more than two people. It can be two-
girls-one-guy, two-guys-one-girl, a couples' swap, or a group orgy situation. Lots of people fantasize about bringing another person (or
two) into the bedroom. It's a way to spice things up for long-term
couples, explore a same-sex erotic experience for a partner who's bi-
sexual or bi-curious, or live out a scene that usually tops the list of ultimate fantasies among straight men. And for women, the idea of
having four hands working at once on them has a great deal of erotic
appeal as well.

Many of the Vivid Girls have fantasized about threesomes, and
they've also had the chance to act them out on film and, sometimes, in
their private lives. "I'm looking forward to trying two guys on film,"

says Mercedez. "I've never done a threesome with a guy and a girl either, so I am excited to give that a try on film, too. Two guys sounds interesting to me, just because watching it turns me on, so I think doing it will be fun, too," she adds. Tawny confesses, "Before I was in the industry, I never even considered a threesome, but now that I have done it, it definitely turns me on and I have done it off camera, too. I think it's a way to shake things up, and I would rather have a threesome than discover my partner cheating."

Sharing one's partner with someone else crosses a lot of boundaries. Savanna says, "Threesomes are very important in my life right now, but it took a while to be able to be cool with it. I was always jealous before. I was a good Catholic girl, so it was difficult for me to be okay with it for myself. When we have other partners, we both want each other to be there. I am amazed my husband is so open. He's even into seeing me with another guy; the thrill of watching me is exciting to him."

There are several issues to consider before embarking on a ménage à trois. First, communicate openly and honestly with your partner about your motivations. Ask yourself and each other why you want to have a threesome. You should never add another person to the mix to fix a failing relationship, or if you feel pressured by your partner to do it. Briana has participated in group scenes on film. In her feature *Swoosh,* for example, she wears a strap-on dildo and joins other couples engaged in various sex acts who are scattered around a swanky, private swimming pool. But in her personal life, she's more of a one-man woman: "I prefer just one-on-one, but that's me," says Briana. "I like to concentrate on one thing at a time. I've had practice and I'm pretty good at it, but for my private life, I'll stick with just one at a time." Both partners need to be equally enthusiastic and comfortable with the idea in order for it to work. Talk to each other about how you envision the fantasy evening, and what your expectations are. Each of you needs to be prepared to see your partner have sex with another person. If the idea freaks you out, the reality most definitely will not make you happy.

Briana cautions couples to be realistic about their expectations and the feelings they may have afterward: "Make sure that a threesome is what you want to do. I've seen couples who didn't think it through, then afterward, someone is jealous, feels neglected. Make sure your relationship can handle it." Bobby tends to agree. "The quickest way to lose your girl is to force her into something she doesn't want to do. Don't do anything that will hurt your relationship."

If you have a frank, openly communicative relationship, it will be easier to discuss the threesome idea and decide whether or not you'll pursue it if the opportunity presents itself. Either way, it's very important to set ground rules before you set a plan in motion. Perhaps the most important thing is to discuss what feels comfortable for both of you. Some guys love the fantasy of being with two women, but can't handle being one of two guys with a woman they love. Similarly, some women love the idea of bringing another female in, but feel bringing in another man would be too much like cheating. Or, she may like the idea of two guys but not be keen on having sex with another woman. Once you've both agreed to try it, you need to decide on the gender of the third person, or if you're going to bring in one or more couples.

Next, decide if there are certain acts—like kissing, oral sex, or intercourse—that are off-limits with the other person. You should also consider whether you want the tryst to happen in your bed or at your house; whether the third person should sleep over; or whether this is something the two of you do on vacations only. By having boundaries, you can both feel more secure that even while getting wild and crazy with your third person, you are still honoring your commitment to each other. As Briana says, "You have to be very comfortable with each other and know that the person you are with is someone you love. After the third person leaves, you're still going to be together. Just because there is another person there doesn't change the way you feel for each other."

Speaking of commitment, make one and reinforce it with each other. Remember that a threesome can be a once-only situation, or recreational fun every now and then. Whichever the case, you need to renew your commitment to each other, and not go running off with the other person. Reassure each other as Briana suggests: "Having boundaries is the most important thing. If either one of the partners thinks what they are doing is wrong, that person is going to get jealous. When I go to work and have sex with someone other than my boyfriend, I know that everything will return to normal after whatever it is I do on camera is done. Having a threesome is like that, too. You have to say, 'Honey, I love you. Let's try this, but if it doesn't work, it's not going to change anything between us.'"

Once your ground rules are established, you have to select your third person. It's a good idea to have some limits about this as well. Some couples agree on certain guidelines like: no coworkers, no neighbors, no close friends, or no one either of you knew before. For a one-time-only event, you may want to consider hiring your third consenting adult by calling one of the escort services listed under the "personal services" section of your local paper. Having a threesome will take plenty of coordination, and you don't want the extra anxiety of worrying about this person making off with the family silver. In order for both people to feel comfortable before, during, and after, make sure you can trust the person to be discreet and respectful of your relationship. Gossips, drama queens, home wreckers, and people with a history of emotional or psychological problems do not make good threesome candidates! "My boyfriend and I would love to pick up another girl, but we're not sure who or where," says Sunrise. Savanna knows other dancers from her days as a stage performer, and often meets them at clubs. She invites them to dinner with her and her husband. Or she and her guy "swing" with other couples in the adult industry. She also likes to surprise her guy: "I think the best surprise for him is to have a girl just show up at the door. Or I'll say, 'I have a surprise for you tonight . . . Someone's coming over.' " To be on the safe side with one or more people you don't really know, meeting at a hotel is a good bet.

> ❝ **The first time that I did have a threesome, it was so wonderful to have someone going down on me and have someone kissing me at the same time.** ❞
>
> —*Savanna*

During a threesome, the focus tends to shift from one person to another to the other. The three-way dynamic is different from the two-sided interaction you are used to. Perhaps your fantasy scenario resembles scenes in *Nurses* or *Student Body* in which two guys make it with one girl. In this combination, usually the girl gives one guy a blow job while the other guy fucks her or goes down on her. Then the guys switch places, or, the action might end up as double penetration. If your fantasy is more like the scene in *Rolling Thunder,* with one guy and two girls, the women are usually more active. One makes her pussy available to his mouth, while the other goes down on him, leaving his hands free to stimulate both of them. Or, the guy penetrates one girl while she manually stimulates and goes down on the other girl. For the finale, a lot depends on how flexible and creative the three of you are. One of many steamy scenes in *Swoosh* culminates in an exciting visual, with one girl sitting Reverse Cowgirl style on the other while the guy alternately penetrates the two of them. The same scenario happens in *Bangkok Nights.*

A particularly hot group scene with many variations between one guy (the writer) and two girls (the stalker and the pickup) takes place in *Obsession.* First the stalker orders the pickup to masturbate with a dildo while she herself is being orally serviced by Jack, the writer. In the next clip, the pickup still uses the dildo while Jack tweaks the pickup's nipples and gets head from the stalker. Then it switches again so that the stalker first uses a dildo in the pickup's ass, and then penetrates her anally with a strap-on. Next, Jack fucks the pickup in the ass while the stalker uses her hands to simultaneously stimulate the pickup's pussy and ass. And, finally, the action ends with the stalker slapping the pickup's ass really hard while at the same time helping Jack masturbate to orgasm.

As in the above, another scenario to consider for threesomes and groups is the use of toys. Dasha masterfully illustrates this in the beginning of *The Vision,* where she and another model are partying with the two dot-commers. She uses a dildo on the other girl while giving one guy head and getting fucked by the second guy.

Bobby offers an important tip for men considering threesomes. "My advice to the guy who wants to try it is, give his girl most of the attention but still give the other girl pleasure, so that your wife or girlfriend still feels more important than that other girl." He also suggests that it may be a good idea to have the third girl do the "more forbidden" things so that your girlfriend or wife feels secure enough to do them if she wants to, and can proceed at her own pace.

It goes without saying that if you are introducing another person into your sex life, you should practice safer sex. Men should use condoms, and change them for different partners. You might also consider latex gloves and oral sex barriers, especially if your third is a total stranger.

After your romp, be ready to talk about it and be prepared if bad feelings and emotions come up. Savanna had to work through some of her issues: "You have to be okay with yourself and secure in your relationship to be okay with having outside partners. He used to say, 'I'd like to see you kiss another woman,' and I couldn't get past [the idea] that he wanted 'her.' It was important for me to realize that doing the threesome or sharing your man with another woman is not him wanting to be with just her. He wants to see me with her. That helped me get past some of my jealousy."

Girl-on-Girl

❝ Having sex with another woman transformed my sexuality. I learned so many new techniques from other women about what feels good. And having a woman do me with a strap-on is a big turn-on for me. ❞

—Tawny

There are plenty of movies that feature girl-on-girl scenes because they are such big turn-ons for men and women alike. Guys get turned on by watching sexed-up girls get down and dirty. And women get turned on because they can relate to all the various sensations each girl is feeling. There is no doubt that women have intimate knowledge about what another woman might like, how to do it well, and how long it will take her. And, as Briana says, "Women are softer, and more lovey-dovey." It stands to reason that they would be curious about touching another woman's breasts, or tasting her clit and pussy. Besides, sometimes a woman just craves a gentler touch, or one that doesn't necessarily end in penetration. "I love a good girl-girl scene," says Sunrise. "I love when a girl is as into you as you are into her. It makes the whole experience very erotic for me."

Movies like *Where the Boys Aren't 14* and *Where the Boys Aren't 15* are chock full of girl-on-girl and all-girl orgy scenes. And the futuristic thriller *Domination Nation* has, as its premise, a world where men are scarce and women are left to satisfy one another. Except for the obvious anatomical differences, there's not much that a man and a woman can do that two women can't do together, especially when they add toys into the mix. "For some reason, two women fooling around isn't as threatening to guys as the idea of you seeing another man," notes Jenna. "Some guys just want to be able to watch, or they just want to hear about it later."

Besides the usual tasting and touching, there are other things that women can do with one another that would be difficult for a man and woman to do with a penis and balls in the way. In *Suite 18,* for example, the women rub their clits and pussies together with their legs crisscrossing each other. And in *Obsession,* there's some energetic dry humping and clit rubbing between the stalker and the pickup girl. Girl-on-girl routines certainly don't replace men, they merely offer a sexual alternative. Savanna says, "When I'm going down on the girl, I love to play with her clit. I just think about what it must feel like, and I get so wet just trying to make her come. I also love to use a double dildo with another woman; we slide each end inside ourselves, and we can rub our clits together. It feels good to be penetrated and also have the girl's pussy against mine."

Briana, however, raises a point about women possibly being more self-conscious about their bodies with another woman. "I didn't really expect that a woman could make me come, or that I would've been turned on by a woman as much as I was when I first started experimenting," she says. "I have more confidence in myself now that I have been with women. You learn to relax and enjoy their beauty and your beauty and not worry about the differences between you. You learn to enjoy your own body more so you can enjoy another woman, too."

Waxing Poetic

Years ago, one didn't hear too much about dripping hot wax on someone as a turn on. But once Madonna did it in a mainstream movie, the idea became more accepted. For some, the turn-on is the fleeting burning sensation made by dripping small amounts of hot wax onto the skin. The temperature of the wax is minimally controlled by the height from which it is dripped. The higher up, the longer it has to reach its destination, and the more it will cool before it touches the skin. For those who enjoy this, one of the big pleasures it touches upon is the "master—slave" relationship. The dripper controls the situation, while the drippee is excited about not knowing when and where the next drop will fall. In *Blondage,* the two star strippers make good use of dripping hot wax on each other as part of their act. And in *Looking In,* the candle-wax visual is pushed a little further. The wife masturbates with one unlit candle inside her vagina and another in her rectum, then her husband lights them. In addition to the sexy visual image, this adds the bondage element of her not being able to move until he removes them. Needless to say, if you try this, you have to be very careful. You don't want to burn someone else, and you don't want to set the house on fire. In *Blondage,* the strippers drip wax from candles inside long glasses. And in *Looking In,* the couple uses very long, formal dinner tapers.

Light Bondage

While Vivid films never depict women in violent or physically abusive situations, some of the films feature light bondage. Bobby tries to shed some light on the psychology of this. "I can't explain it," he says. "I want to have something that I do that another other guy is not going to do. I'll just grab her, push her up against the wall, and start kissing her and kissing her. She'll be transported to another place, and suddenly you're the warrior and she's the captive. All the rough stuff is about sending you to that place. It's got a certain ritual to it, and it's all about the forbidden."

A very tongue-in-cheek illustration of light bondage takes place in *Domination Nation,* in which "the year is 6969, and justice is a bitch!" In this future world, men die immediately after ejaculation, so they flee the ruling "glamazons," who force them to have sex. In one scene, the Alpha Woman and her disciple catch a man by shooting him with a stun gun, and then bind his struggling body in chains. The image of the long-haired hunk struggling to break his chains brings to mind the Greek myth about Prometheus chained to the rock, or the biblical story of Samson, who was brought before the palace court in chains. It's very sexy to imagine such a hottie bound up to do one's bidding.

A little more down-to-earth is the bondage scene between the two leads in *Jenna Loves Rocco*. In addition to the chains, whips, and other props on the wall, Jenna wears a kinky-looking bra made of chains, black patent-leather opera-length gloves, and black patent-leather panties with garters on her stockings. First she handcuffs Rocco's wrists, then she climbs on top of him, teases him mercilessly, and removes her clothing so they can finally have sex. The action culminates with her removing the wrist restraints, and leading him over to a black leather sling, where he forcefully pulls her hair back and fucks her. Later in the scene, she pleads with him to hurt her. Realizing that she wants to go further than he does, Rocco makes his getaway.

Occasional light bondage, including handcuffs and the like, has made its way into the mainstream. More serious aficionados tend to frequent special parties and clubs, but that's a much more involved scenario than a couple who just want to experiment with the "me Tarzan, you Jane" fantasy. The rule of thumb when engaging in this sort of thing is that there should always be a safe word or signal, *agreed upon beforehand,* which lets the other person know it's time to stop the action.

Fetishes

Most fetishes are totally harmless, and can add a little twist to things from time to time. One such fetish can be seen in *Obsession,* for example, where the stalker rubs a photo of the writer against her clit to masturbate. High heels, thigh-high stiletto boots, and lacy thongs are all staples in the costume department of the adult film industry. In *Where the Boys Aren't 14,* however, these props are used as part of the action as well as for decoration. At one point, Dasha has another girl lick her boots and suck on the high heel. Later, she uses the boot's pointy toe to massage the other girl's pussy, then was the heel to rip off the girl's panties. Fetishes to do with shoes and boots are among the most common. Other clothing fetishes include dressing up in costume or uniforms such as cops, nurses, schoolgirls, and cowboys. Still others are linked to particular fabrics or textures, such as leather, satin, or latex. (See Chapter 13 for "Vivid Girl Favorites: Secret Fantasies.")

There are also those who get turned on by feet without the boots or shoes. Toe sucking, or a guy inserting his toe into a girl's pussy, is fairly common and mainstream. But in *One Way Out* and *The Most Beautiful Girl in the World,* feet take on a bigger role. These films include scenes of the woman masturbating the guy with the soles of her feet, and of the girl asking the guy to come on her feet. The soft, arched underside of the foot can make this a very sensual experience for both parties involved.

Fetishes that are a bit kinkier require mutual agreement on who does what to whom, when, and how, especially for those that involve B&D (bondage and discipline) or S&M (sadism and masochism). In *Blondage,* such fetishes are used as part of the girl-on-girl club act. At one point, both girls wear black leather masks. At another point, one girl slowly spanks the other's bottom so that it gets a rosy glow. They take this further by swinging a small cat-o'-nine-tails, implying a slave-and-master relationship. This fantasy is carried even further when one girl leads the other around by a dog collar and leash, and when she harnesses the other girl with a horse bit and reins, and rides her around the stage.

Similarly, a model dressed in chains and chained to a spiderweb contraption is part of an artist's performance piece in *Jenna Loves Rocco.* As part of the performance, the artist directs the woman and another male model to touch each other and have sex a certain way. There's also a scene in the performance where a girl has a stick inserted up her pussy. In the big sex-party scene in *Obsession,* a girl is harnessed into a bottomless metal seat so that her pussy and clit are exposed for others to lick. As with all such activities, fetish activity requires excellent communication and understanding of one's partner's fantasies, a high level of trust, and, sometimes, a sense of humor.

15
a star is porn

You know the old cliché of the bachelor pad with the mirror on the ceiling above the bed? Well, it may be obvious, but watching yourself have sex can be quite a turn on. The modern technological equivalent of the mirror on the ceiling is the camcorder by the bed.

One of the reasons why people watch adult videos is to see activities they may not get to experience in their real lives. That's because many movies feature fantasies and elements of a sexual world beyond the norm. In adult movies, one sees people with unique abilities, not to mention performers who are exceedingly attractive, perfectly groomed, and have fabulous bodies to boot! And what's really nice about these films is that you can play your favorite scene over and over again. If you've ever watched a porn movie, seen something alternative, racy, or wild, and thought, "Hey, I want to try that!" then this chapter is for you.

If you have exhibitionist tendencies, then watching yourself on film can be a real turn-on. Turn on the VCR, pop in a video, and make love with your own personal porno playing in the background. You can also use it to improve your skills as a lover. Tawny compares it to professional ballplayers watching a game at practice: "Watch it and critique each other, tell him what worked and what didn't. Give him some pointers for next time. Of course, you can just watch to get off on it or do both!"

❝ ❝ I think it's great when couples make their own videos if they are both into it. It's great to watch yourselves afterward, and you'll have plenty of masturbation material for later. ❞ ❞

—*Savanna*

Today, more people than ever have video cameras. Many even have special software to view and edit their creations on the computer as well as the ability to add a sound track. But you really don't need lots of high-tech equipment; a camcorder and a tripod will work fine. And if you want to add Wagner, Keith Jarrett, or 50 Cent as background music to your moans and sighs, just turn on the stereo while you're taping.

Briana has another, more upscale spin on the homemade tape. "There are places now that make home videos for couples," she says. "You go, do your thing, and they get all the angles. They give you the master tape. I recommend that because then you don't have to worry about any technical stuff." And, if you're concerned about what happens to the tapes later (remember Pamela Anderson and Tommy Lee's homemade video? Or the Paris Hilton video circulating on the Internet?), take care to erase them.

One note of caution: once you're on tape, there's always the possibility that, one day, someone might unexpectedly see your video. If you have kids and want to keep your recording for posterity, it's a good idea to put the tape someplace where they'll never discover it—preferably in a locked box. Similarly, the Internet is filled with photos and videos of former girlfriends (and boyfriends) in compromising positions. So you really have to trust your partner and establish the rules. Another idea is to set up the camcorder without any tape in it at all. Just plug the camera into the TV so you can watch yourselves in real time.

Prepping the Set

Speaking of rules, Paul points out that the most important preparations for making a video go beyond the obvious romantic lighting and proper music. "Two people have to ask themselves what they want out of this evening," he says. "Do they want intimacy between the two of them, or are they looking for some extracurricular additive to the evening? Do they expect a whole cast of characters to show up at the door? Is the busboy invited up? Do you open the curtains for the neighbors to peer in? Are they looking for a special twist or kink for the evening?" Prepping the stage means discussing all of this with your partner so you both know what you're getting into, and won't be disappointed. "What's always most fun is what's spontaneous,"

SPECIALTIES

Savanna: "My thing to do is sucking cock because I love it so much. I want to please him so badly. I love the way it feels in my mouth, and I love the feel of it in my hands."

Briana: "Blow jobs! I have no gag reflex. I never knew I had this specialty because all of my previous boyfriends were very small. And it wasn't until I was in the 'biz' that deep throating became possible. I'm also known for my anal scenes; and I really enjoy doing it."

Dasha: "I guess the squirting thing."

Sunrise: "My specialty would have to be blow jobs. I learned on a banana!"

Kira: "Double penetration!"

Jenna: "It would definitely have to be blow jobs!"

Paul continues. "So if they have something special in mind they have to provide for it. Otherwise, just allow for the time and space and privacy that's needed, and let it happen. To plan things out too precisely can kill it. And to have overly specific expectations can kill it unless, of course, they've agreed on things long beforehand."

Bobby tends to agree with Paul. "It's pretty important to have an understanding that whatever may happen that evening is by virtue of mutual consent so that there are no recriminations after the fact.

If you set up a video camera, and that's something you normally wouldn't do, maybe that would be even 'dirtier' than following someone into the bathroom."

Be Your Own Porn Star

❝ ❝ Videotaping yourselves can be a very naughty thing. ❞ ❞

—Bobby

Bobby enjoys this immensely with his partner because, at home, he finds it the complete opposite of being on a movie set. "If we're in a kinky mood, I like to put the camera on us and plug it into the big-screen TV," says Bobby. "We see ourselves raw and real and right there—live. If we're in a kinky mood, I'm going to point the camera right at the couch. Sometimes we'll be laughing, or we'll do it so hard, we'll knock the camera right off the shelf. But keeping it real and raw is what it's all about."

"Anything you try for the first time, try to get comfortable, open your mind, and don't be pigheaded. Just enjoy it." says Briana. "You only get one first time for something, so don't waste it. With me, my first time for so many things is all on film, so I can go back and savor it."

From Set to Bedroom

Maybe you've noticed that the gorgeous Vivid Girls look perfectly made up and coiffed for their scenes? Well, that's because, as with all quality film productions, there are makeup artists and hairstylists to help the performers look their very best. You may not want to ask your hairdresser to stand by while you're taping at home, but you might want to think about your makeup and clothing—if you plan on wearing any.

By all means, this is the perfect time to pull out the fishnet hose and stilettos, the "merry widow," or the frilliest fuchsia bra-and-thong set. If you don't have any "specialty items" you'd like to wear, watch some videos to see what the Vivid Girls are wearing. Usually, the clothes are stylish and sexy, but not outrageous. The same goes for the guys. If you got turned on by *Lotus,* maybe you could find kimonos like the ones worn by the Emperor and the concubine? If you liked *Student Body,* it shouldn't be too hard to scrounge up a football jersey and a cheerleading sweater. And if your longtime fantasy involves nurses and doctors, any uniform store will have inexpensive "costumes" to help you realize it.

Once you and your partner have decided to capture yourselves on tape, the next thing to determine is if you'll do your usual routine or try something new. We asked Team Vivid what they thought people would try because they saw it in a porn movie. Mercedez says, "I think people will try creative positions," while Kira opts

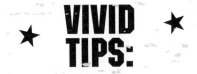

VIVID TIPS:

★ VIVID TIPS: ★

VIVID TIPS: HOW TO KEEP A LONG-TERM RELATIONSHIP HOT

Mercedez: "I've been with the same guy for eight years, and I think the best thing is his attitude. He is always willing to try new things. He's open to toys, and we just started getting into anal sex. I know I could come to him with an idea, fantasy, and he'd be up for it."

Kira: "Remember to keep dating even after you've been together for a while. Dress up for each other, go out, flirt like you did when you first met."

Briana: "Keep it exciting, be spontaneous—you don't want your partner hopping the fence to the neighbor's house."

Tawny: "Try having sex in unexpected places or even semipublic places. Change it up, try the unexpected."

Jenna: "I don't always like knowing when we're going to have sex. I love it when he's spontaneous, like if we are getting ready to go somewhere, and I am blow-drying my hair. He comes up to me, and I'm caught off guard. It's hot."

for "double penetration." "People's big fascinations are things like being doubled, or doing a blow job with your head hanging off the side of a table," says Briana. "Some things people are never going to experience, and they are just a great fantasy; others are going to give it a try," she adds. Jenna and Dasha both say "anal sex," with Dasha adding "sex with more than one person; or sex with women."

Sunrise puts things quite eloquently: "It depends on what a couple is looking for—a new position, or how to tie up your lover," she says. "Growing up, I was one of those people watching movies and learning from them. I used to love watching movies and trying new positions. The best thing would just be to explore and try different things, and then be open-minded enough to try it. Don't be afraid of it just because it's new or different. Even today, I see a new position and I want to try it. I use porn to guide me along."

Of course, sometimes you have to be prepared to discover

that the fantasy you had in mind may not be as heavenly as you thought. Briana recounts an incident in front of the camera when one of her fantasies didn't turn out quite as she expected. "I've pretty much acted all the fantasies I had, and even ones I didn't know I had. For me, I've pretty much experienced everything. But the fantasy I had about being with girls didn't quite turn out as I had envisioned it. I had the whole thing with the milk and roses with Dasha in the bathtub. But the milk was freezing cold! It was one of those things that was better as a fantasy than as a reality. I was so cold! It was fun, but . . . I'd much rather be really hot and have to do a scene than be shaking and my lips are blue. I really get cold easily."

Postproduction

When the two of you have finished what you're going to do, what you do after can be as important to your relationship as what you did during the act. You don't stop loving each other just because you're now lying side by side in a pool of sweat.

Chances are you'll both be somewhat gooey and sticky by now, with lube, natural fluids, and sweat. Some people keep a supply of small towels near their bed for cleanup purposes. If you remember one of the tips Mercedez learned on the set, try a container of unscented baby wipes for easy cleaning. If you really want to give your partner the star treatment, bring him or her a washcloth wet with warm water from the tap. If you're both not too tired and your legs aren't so jellylike that you can't stand, you can take a shower together.

Sometimes you're lying there in each other's arms, and neither of you is quite sleepy yet. And you start to talk. Sometimes it just happens, but this is an intimate time when you can learn a lot about each other. You may find out things you would never find out in a thousand dinner conversations. Now is the time to bring up any ideas you'd like to reinforce, such as "I really liked it when you did that thing with your tongue . . ." or gentle suggestions for next time.

Now is not the time to criticize, however—let any serious lapses that were not brought up already during the action wait until the morning (but don't wait too long and definitely bring it up before the next date). And thank your lover before you drift off to sleep for costarring in your fabulous erotic production.

Vivid Entertainment

Details magazine called Vivid Entertainment "the Microsoft of the porn industry," the biggest and most widely known of all adult film companies. Over the years, Vivid has grown into the top adult company through a strong commitment to quality product. As far as the adult film industry goes, Vivid is truly unique. Not only do the films have attractive stars and high-quality production values, but they also have been characterized as "couples-friendly porn for the thinking person." In other words, most of the scripts have complex plots, good character development, and psychological insights into what is erotic for the twenty-first century man and woman. The characters are ones to which everyday people can easily relate: doctors, lawyers, students, taxi drivers, businesspeople, neighbors, and even a girl doing her laundry in the basement of her apartment building. Moreover, the films emphasize nonviolent, consensual relationships between attractive, articulate people.

Much of Vivid's philosophy has been shaped by its founders. But the people who put these ideas into practice are the directors. Here are some of their stories, "Up Close & Personal":

Paul Thomas, Director

Paul Thomas, or PT as he is known, began his career as an actor and performer on Broadway, appearing in shows like *Jesus Christ Superstar* and *Hair,* and in mainstream television shows like *Mannix* and *Police Story.* In the "swinging seventies" era of "porn chic," he switched to the adult industry and starred in over four hundred movies. "Did you see the movie *Boogie Nights*?" PT asks. "That was the story of my life." PT never felt he abandoned his original professional goals. Going into adult movies "wasn't a compromise," he says. "I was a hippie then. It was an extension of my swinging lifestyle."

At thirty-five, PT turned to directing, and has been the auteur-in-residence for Vivid since 1986. His adult movies feature such strong character elements and intriguing plots that he also films R-rated versions of them. "I'm expected to go beyond the obvious," PT says of his never-ending search for originality. "The couple looking for something new has the same challenge we do in films. You want it to seem completely spontaneous, but at the same time you have to plan for it, and be prepared for it."

PT has been directing adult movies for a long time; long enough to see the business veer from expensive film productions to amateur and home videos, and back to the high-quality movies he directs now for Vivid. "I'm known as the king of 'couples' films," he says, and for making movies that have engaging characters and intriguing sexual action beyond the usual adult fare. With Vivid's high standards, choreographing a sex scene for film is much like choreographing a dance sequence or even a fight scene. "Some of my most successful films are the ones where the sex scenes are written out, from beginning to end. It's so necessary to direct some of the professionals; otherwise it's so predictable that even I can't watch it."

The films PT directs for Vivid reflect his own aesthetic sensibility, often depicting sexual acts that are considered fairly common for today's couples. "In my films, people aren't performing for the camera, they're doing the same things they would do if they were in their living rooms. Sure, the actors are putting on a show for the camera in that I want them to show what they're doing. But some people's sexual preferences are too intimate for the camera's taste. Apart from the stories I tell in the movies, my job is to have people be as seductive and attractive to each other for as long as possible without having sex." This is where good directing comes in. "I coach them, and encourage them to tease, to take as long as possible, and be as sexual with each other as possible, but to try to put off intercourse for as long as possible. And just because they've started, doesn't mean they have to continue to climax. There are other erotic things that they can do besides have intercourse. The more interactive people are, the more interesting it will be to watch."

In the same way that the adult film world has drastically changed over the years, so has PT's own sex life. "I had been involved in a lot of group-sex situations, but since AIDS, since HIV, it's no fun anymore. I think I've had enough anonymous sex. I'm exclusively intimate with one woman now, and I want to stay that way—but I can make that statement because I've had so much sex. Now I'm really starting to explore intimacy. I'm starting to look for the excitement and intimacy without the mention of anything kinky. Just two people together, because it's been absent from my life for so long—now, *that* to me is kinky."

The adult film industry is fueled by the power of fantasy. PT's interest in fantasy and the suspension of disbelief is a quality that makes his movies successful. But the same factors affect his personal life, too. It's something he's thought about a lot. "When you're in a relationship, it's difficult to be original and creative when you, invariably, begin to repeat the same words and phrases." Does this mean that PT thinks sex exclusively between two people is doomed to be boring? "Not unless you have low expectations," he says. He loves the idea of using fantasy to keep the fires burning in a relationship.

"I have a philosophy about fantasies," he says. "I think fantasies need enough fuel to make them exciting. Once in a while you need to make them real, so it's necessary to personalize them. Just once in a blue moon, you have to 'bring other people and events in,' and interact with them. But you don't really have to have sex with them," PT continues. "You tease, tell stories. You want your partner to have suspension of disbelief long enough to arouse them. I'm still encouraging my partner to talk to me about men or women she 'sees,' and lie to me while I'm aroused about some outrageous situation that happened to her today that, for the time being, I buy into."

And what are some of PT's favorite personal fantasies? "I am obsessed with thinking about and seeing the woman that I care for—and I have to care for her—with another man. She can tell me about other adventures she's had, or we can go out and she can pick up or tease another man. And I love sex in public places, where people are watching who shouldn't be watching. That's been my 'fantasy' thing for a long time."

PT's work focuses on giving form to fantasies on film. But how does he see this working between two people in real life? "Fantasies are very powerful. Sex is very powerful. It takes honest communication to make it work," states PT. "The worst thing in the world is when one person levels blame or anger at the other partner, whether it's the next morning, two weeks later, or a year later. It has to be mutual." Experience has taught him to check with his partner, and then check with her again to make sure she is okay with the fantasies they play with. "It's pretty important to have an understanding that whatever may happen that evening is by virtue of mutual consent so that there are no recriminations after the fact. My favorite bent is to see the woman I care for teasing, sometimes touching, or being touched by another man. I've gotten into situations where the evening would take off, and the woman was very turned on by the idea which we discussed at length beforehand, and was very turned on while it was happening, but I would get it thrown back in my face the next morning or the next week. How could I compromise her virtue in such a way? Maybe a written agreement isn't such a bad idea," he muses.

PT cautions that people shouldn't feel guilty about a less-than-perfect performance, or being "sex stars" all the time. "It's not good to force it if you're not feeling it. And if two people end up on two ends of the spectrum at the conclusion of an evening, maybe they weren't right for each other in the first place."

Now that he's older, PT finds it easier to maintain a healthy balance in his sex life, and the place of sex in his life. "One has to decide for oneself what place sex should take in one's life—the proper level, the amount of your energy that it needs to take," he says. "In my experience, if sex seems to be just consuming you, then it's not healthy; it's not going to lead to good relationships or personal satisfaction. It needs to be treated with respect and with balance in the rest of your life."

He is philosophical about the importance of sex in a relationship as well. "If these sessions, these evenings we're speaking of in this book, don't seem to work, maybe the answer, rather than ditching the relationship, is to just forget the evening. Sex doesn't have to be such a huge part of your life. If it's not flowing, if it's not happening, rather than losing the relationship, maybe you should consider lessening the importance of sex in the relationship."

In today's world of readily available images in the media and on the Internet, PT, as a well-respected adult film director, has been asked to appear on TV shows, especially when the topic of the day is the sex and the porn industry. "I've been on talk shows where the topic is 'Is Porn Addicting?' he says. "They expect me to say 'no, it's not,' and I've said 'damn straight it's addicting.' But I can't think of hardly anyone who would rather watch a porno movie than watch a Lakers game," he says with a twinkle in his eye.

Chi Chi LaRue, Director

How did a young man named Larry, who grew up in Minnesota and became a six-foot one-inch drag performer, come to direct over a hundred gay male porn videos and end up doing high-budget heterosexual features for Vivid Entertainment? We're not sure, but the fabulous and award-winning Chi Chi LaRue brings something fresh and different to every movie production.

Even in college, Chi Chi was a connoisseur of classic porn. "I read *Cinema Blue* like the Bible. And in my art classes, I made a collage of women I loved, and right in the middle was [adult movie star] Marilyn Chambers."

As a gay man, Chi Chi brings a unique perspective to straight sex and often makes suggestions to his straight actors that straight directors might not think of. He sees making quality porn films as a form of public service: "I want people to have fun sex," he says. "I wouldn't want anyone to watch a porn movie if it offends them." Chi Chi also speculates on why his films are so popular with straight couples: "As I go on directing these movies, I learn a lot about straight sex. Sure, a woman's breasts are important to the look of the film, but I found that if you have a good amount of focus on the guy, the film will appeal more to women." And Chi Chi feels his films are educational as well. "If you can watch a porn movie and get some tips from the performers, then that's great," he says. "They are a tool you can use to stay home and pleasure yourself, or to enhance your sex life with a partner. Watching a film is safe, especially Vivid films," he continues. "Their policies on safe sex and the use of condoms in every movie show people how to have sex responsibly."

By his own admission, Chi Chi is a director who tends to talk a lot on the set. So it stands to reason that one of the "hot and safe" things he considers a turn-on is the use of dirty talk. "Sometimes I just whisper something dirty in a performer's ear and it will speed things along," he says. "Besides, you can be having normal, vanilla sex in one position, go a little crazy and say something dirty, and you're off in another world. You can say lots of nasty things that you'd never do!"

Chi Chi says he is often impressed by the acrobatic feats his actors achieve. "An adult movie is about creating amazing visuals, so the scenarios are often bizarre—like sex in an alley or hanging on some sawhorses or on a ladder—things most people don't do at home. I did a scene recently with Kody and Lee Stone where he picks her up, and they have sex while he's holding her in the air. I shot Troy Halston and Holly Halston when he held her up and went down on her. That's acrobatics! I don't know how many people can physically do that in their bedroom, but it certainly enhances the visual effect for the camera!"

Beyond the acrobatic feats, Chi Chi has nothing but admiration for his performers. "The payoff of my job is working with women who love what they do. Working with someone like Jenna Jameson is so worth it. I did a scene with Jenna and Dasha and they just did their thing, they didn't even really need a lot of direction. Once I filmed a certain scene with Briana Banks and Bobby Vitale, and Briana just rocked!"

And the guys? "Keeping it hard on the set is definitely a challenge. But there are so many performers, like Dillon Day and Dale DeBone, who are hard from the second a scene starts. It just doesn't go down; and it keeps going—which is brilliantly amazing. That's why there are so many tried-and-true performers; you don't have to worry about 'wood' problems."

Chi Chi is always looking for performers who will push the envelope a little with him. "I like when straight couples explore anal sex. I think it's an area where some straight couples rarely go. I know some people think it's a little bit of a control or dominant kind of feeling when a well-endowed man is having anal sex with a woman." Sometimes they're in one position or another, "and I'm so concerned about how the girl is feeling, I'm biting my finger. Are they hating this? But they're loving it. And it impresses everyone—cast and crew alike. And for a woman to do it to a man, it's so unexplored, and I think it's the hottest!"

But there are areas Chi Chi is not interested in exploring. Wild as his films are, they are never violent. "I film dirty, dirty sex, but I don't cross the line. I film stuff that couples can actually do or fantasize about doing. Sure, a little hair pulling can be sexy, but that's about as far as I like it to go. I never want to shoot any sex that looks hateful, or that's degrading to the people involved."

And what's the best part about being one of the premier directors of hot movies? "The porn world itself is so small, and everybody knows everybody else's business. What's really refreshing is when you get to work with a new guy or a new girl, and they are so excited to do a sex scene. Their enthusiasm means they have the best scene! When people honestly enjoy having sex with their costars, it makes my job easy and lots of fun."

Justin Sterling, Director

Justin leads the pack of the young generation of adult movie producers. With an eye for beauty and a taste for intriguing images, this award-winning director likes to work his own camera. Named one of the "50 Most Powerful Men Under 37" by *Details* magazine, Justin is also an Internet entrepreneur and cofounder of ClubJenna.com with Jenna Jameson. Justin and Jenna are not only a great pair in business, but are also partners in life. After more than four years together, they were married in 2003 and have plans to raise a family. "He's one of the most sexually free people I've ever known," Jenna says of her mate.

Justin Sterling's entrepreneurial spirit originally drew him to the adult industry. His friend Michael Ninn, then an adult movie editor, and now an award-winning director, asked Justin to invest in a film. Because he didn't know anything about porn movies, Justin decided to work in production on the set in order to learn more about the industry. He worked his way up, then started producing and directing his own films.

Over seven years ago, Justin met Jenna Jameson when she arrived at his studio to shoot a movie. "I thought she was young and bratty, a little arrogant and standoffish, and she didn't like me." Three years later, the pair ran into each other at a party hosted by Playboy, where performer/director Jill Kelly played matchmaker, encouraging each one about the other. "I went up to her, grabbed her, and dragged her out of the party. We both tried to keep it under wraps that we were dating because we talked shit about each other for years. But we were photographed together at a restaurant, then [Jenna's publicist at the time] Joy King and everyone at Wicked Pictures found out. We moved to Arizona shortly after that."

So what brought these two former adversaries together? "In terms of physical attraction, eyes drive me," says Justin. "Jenna has the sexiest eyes on earth; they are the window to her soul. She can project any emotion she wants through her eyes, and they make me melt! Her lips, mouth, a little swipe of the tongue now and then can really drive me wild." But the interior of a person is very important, too. "I need someone who is very open-minded and caring, someone who has confidence and a good sense of humor. I want to be with someone who is happy for other people when something good happens instead of being jealous. And of course, I like someone who's a little bratty, devilish, and playful."

Justin is very traditional when it comes to how to treat a woman: "There are things that women absolutely notice. Be a gentleman—open the door, pull out her chair, don't start eating before she does, help her in and out of the car, stand up when she stands up. Manners are more impressive than anything on a date. Every girl I have ever dated has complimented me on it. Jenna and I knew each other for a while, but when we went out on out first date, I was all about manners. I went to Catholic school, and my parents made me read Emily Post, so I know how to behave."

Justin is cofounder of Jenna's official website, clubjenna.com, and directs many of Jenna's feature films for Vivid. Because they work together, it's a challenge sometimes to separate work and play. "I think it's really important in any relationship to make time for each other away from work, you have to have a balance. But that's even more true with me and Jenna. It's a 24/7 business at our house, and I am definitely a workaholic. I'll work eighty to a hundred hours a week, and then come home and work on the computer. I had to learn that spending time on a plane as we travel is not quality time! So, at our house, each month, we take a four-day break."

Justin says that in the United Kingdom and the rest of Europe, it's the male stars who sell an adult movie, but in the United States, it's the female stars. "Jenna has a big female fan base: 40 to 50 percent," he says. "We look on our website and they post their pictures—they're beautiful." And what does he feel is the role of porn movies in our society? "Watching an adult movie is a great aid to any relationship," he says. "No matter what, sex will become stale in a relationship. You always have to try new things, and you can see a lot of new things in adult movies; it opens you up sexually."

Behind the Scenes: Safer Sex on the Set

Whether you talk nice or dirty, one conversation every couple should have before sex is about practicing safer sex. Vivid Entertainment requires that all actors and actresses use condoms for vaginal and anal intercourse scenes. In addition, Vivid follows adult industry guidelines that require all performers to have current (within thirty days) HIV tests, and a full STD panel. Those new to the industry are tested for syphilis before their first shoot, and everyone must have a syphilis test every six months.

We recommend that you get tested, too, for all sexually transmitted diseases (STDs), including HIV, gonorrhea, chlamydia, syphilis, herpes, human papilloma virus (HPV), genital warts, and hepatitis. If you are in a monogamous relationship, and both of you have tested negative for all STDs, you can do all the things discussed in this book without fear of transmitting any diseases. However, if you have a new sexual partner, are unaware of your partner's STD status and sexual history, or are waiting to be retested, we recommend you practice safer sex. Practicing safer sex means you shouldn't share bodily fluids (like semen, vaginal fluids, menstrual blood, and female ejaculate) with a partner and you should use barriers to protect yourself from infecting your partner, or becoming infected by your partner.

Oral Sex Barriers

Although Vivid doesn't require barriers for oral sex, if you want to practice safe cunnilingus and analingus (rimming), you have several different options. The most popular safe-sex tool for oral-vaginal and oral-anal contact is a square of latex called a dental dam. You can buy them at sex-toy stores; the most popular brand is Glyde Dams, because they are large, superthin, and were designed with this very thing in mind. Some folks prefer plastic wrap (like Saran Wrap) for this kind of play, since it's cheaper, easier to find, and it's clear, so you can see what you are licking! You can also make your own dam out of a rubber (or non-rubber) glove. Cut off the wrist of the glove, then cut up the side where the pinky is, and cut off all four fingers, leaving the thumb intact. Slide your tongue inside the thumb, and you've got the equivalent of a condom for your tongue. Use a little flavored lube on the inside for extra tongue sensitivity. With all oral sex barriers, you should always use lube on the side that faces your partner's genitals to add comfort and sensation as well as reduce friction. (For more on lube, see Chapter 7.)

Rubber Gloves

Vivid also does not require that performers use rubber gloves when using their fingers and hands to stimulate and penetrate one another's orifices. But there are reasons to have gloves on hand: to practice safer sex, to protect a cut or scrape on your hand, or if you and your lover want to play doctor! Some couples also like to use them for anal play, in order to feel confident about their personal hygiene and make cleanup easier. You can buy latex gloves in drugstores and sex-toy stores; at sex-toy stores, you'll often find a much bigger selection, including a variety of sizes, colors, and materials. In this case, size *does* matter: the better the glove fits, the smoother your hand will feel inside your partner and the more feeling and sensitivity you'll have as you try to make them squirm. Always add lubricant to your gloved hand before inserting it into anything. If you or your partner is allergic or sensitive to latex, you can purchase gloves made of vinyl or nitrile.

Condoms

Found on the set of every Vivid film, condoms are an effective way to protect yourself from STDs as well as pregnancy during vaginal and anal intercourse. You can also use condoms on sex toys like vibrators, dildos, and butt plugs, if you are sharing them with another person. The majority of condoms on the market are latex (we'll discuss non-latex varieties shortly) and many come prelubricated. Most prelubricated condoms contain non-oxynol-9 or another spermicide, which can be very irritating to the delicate tissues that make up the vagina and rectum. We suggest choosing nonlubricated condoms, and adding your favorite lube to them (see Chapter 7).

Condoms come in sizes, too, so if your guy is smaller than average, several brands offer a snugger-fitting model. If he's well endowed, you can try longer and larger-size condoms like Durex Maximum, Lifestyles Large, Maxx, and Trojan Large and Magnum. If he's extralarge porn-star size, go for Trojan Magnum XL (a favorite among performers in the adult industry). The biggest complaint about condoms is that they reduce a man's sensitivity, but there are a lot of thinner, stronger condoms on the market now—including Durex Avanti, Beyond Seven, Crown, Kimono, and Trojan Ultra Thin—as well as some new brands like Inspiral and Pleasure Plus that promise greater sensation through inventive design. If you're looking for condoms that actually enhance pleasure, all the major brands have a variety with "bells and whistles." Remember that textures—like bumps, dots, ribbing, ridges, or studs—on the inside of the condom are designed to increase his sensitivity and on the outside are meant to stimulate her. Vivid markets it own line of condoms as well, which includes large size, studded, and extra thin.

Flavored condoms are perfect for blow jobs, and Durex, Impulse, Lifestyles, and Trustex make everything from mint to plum. There are also nonlatex condoms (like Durex Avanti and Trojan Supra, made of polyurethane) if you or your partner is allergic or sensitive to latex. Condoms made of natural lambskin are actually permeable by some STDs, so we don't recommend those for safer sex.

And, remember, a novelty condom is just that—a novelty. So if you received a condom at a bachelor party that's imprinted with something like *Bob's Last Fling,* or if you come across something that has stars and stripes, or a drawing of a Harley on it, it probably hasn't gone through the same inspection that the more popular name brands must pass. In this case, it's preferable to go with a known and trusted source.

Finally, just like food, most condoms have expiration dates printed on the wrapper. Never take a chance on a package that's been opened, and always check for the expiration date. It's better to be safe than sorry.